FREEDOM FROM
CHRONIC DISEASE

FREEDOM FROM
CHRONIC DISEASE

*A Drug-Free Nutritional Program
for Managing Your Health Problems*

Arthur L. Kaslow, M.D., and Richard B. Miles

JEREMY P. TARCHER, INC.
Los Angeles

Distributed by Houghton Mifflin Company
Boston

ACKNOWLEDGMENTS

TO MY ESTEEMED COAUTHOR, RICHARD MILES, MY GRATITUDE
for your unstinting efforts in the search for why our nutritional program is
bearing fruit in gardens declared by others to be barren and therefore
unimportant in the achievement of improvement in health.

And to the innumerable seminar participants and colleagues in the
healing profession who attend the many lectures, seminars, and workshops
as well as personally visit our Medical Centers, for their interest and
professional support of our nutritional self-care concepts and individualized
patient program.

Arthur L. Kaslow, M.D.

Library of Congress Cataloging in Publication Data

Kaslow, Arthur L.
    Freedom from chronic disease.

    Bibliography: p. 267
    Includes index.
    1. Food allergy.   2. Chronic diseases—Nutritional aspects.
3. Nutritionally induced diseases—Prevention.   4. Chronic diseases—
Diet therapy.   5. Self-care, Health.
I. Miles, Richard B.   II. Title.
RC596.K36   1984   613.2'6   83-24256
ISBN 0–87477–318–0

Jeremy P. Tarcher, Inc.
9110 Sunset Blvd.
Los Angeles, CA 90069

Design by Barbara Monahan

Manufactured in the United States of America
    v 10   9   8   7   6   5   4

CONTENTS

Part II   The Kaslow Program

PREFACE TO THE REVISED EDITION

ALTHOUGH THE RESPONSE DIET, THE INDIVIDUAL-FOOD-per-meal testing program we used originally, has proved to be very significant in helping our patients identify foods that are rejected and in signaling symptoms of dysfunction, it is very time-consuming and frustrating to the active and busy person with time limits for self-care. Our experience was that for many of our patients this single-food testing program was proving to be so difficult to carry out that noncompliance and failure on a long-term basis overshadowed the good results that had been accomplished by strict adherence for a short period of time.

Many nurses are patients in our Medical Centers, and during lengthy discussions with them on how to carry out an effective nutritional program, we discovered a practical program of food testing that is a virtual breakthrough in treating nutrigenic diseases.

What we learned by testing an individual food at a single meal was that the quantity of food on the plate was usually sufficiently large to cause a rejectivity response, resulting in an exacerbation of the symptom-signals. Thus, the patients had to eliminate more and more foods from their diets. We were witnessing patients new to the Medical Center who were becoming weak and malnourished—in addition to the symptoms of their original diseases—having been placed on the food rotation diets or the traditional elimination diets. Obviously, this could not be the long-term treatment for certain patients. The anxiety many patients experienced when the number of eliminated foods finally restricted their intake to three or four foods a week turned to panic when they began to react adversely to this rotating diet program. Many patients we saw were already in a state of malnutrition due to chronic food rejectivity or to the elimination of many foods tested individually in a rotating diet program. To prevent this serious deficiency from developing on a long-term basis in the nutritional program, we evolved the 8 Mini-Food Meal program (8 MFM). This program is included at the end of Chapter 8 of this revised edition, as an extension of "A Personal Workbook for Health."

With the 8 MFM program, there seems to be a *total elimination* of the symptom-signals related to the Metabolic Rejectivity Syndrome. The second bonus is the beneficial consequence of eating a wide variety of natural foods. Our patients experience the benefits of supplying the body with a more complete nutritional base for the forty-five nutritional substances needed for the well-being they so eagerly seek. They feel the difference about two weeks after starting the 8 Mini-Food Meal program. Following this program also reduces meal preparation time to a total of two days a week in the kitchen. Our nurse patients and many others with time constraints describe this as a "vacation at home," the best kind!

PREFACE

SINCE THE EARLY 1950s I HAVE BEEN ACCUMULATING evidence that nutrition is the central key in the development and perpetuation of chronic illness, and that balancing the body's natural self-healing processes and supporting the patient's nutritional and psychological needs are major factors in breaking disease cycles. In many of my patients—even those with balanced and essentially nutritious diets—I found a definite relationship between the foods they ate and the recurrence of their disease symptoms. Some "nutritious" foods actually caused adverse reactions.

My startling realization led me to clinical research into the biological individuality of nutrition. This journey eventually led me to the formulation of the "Metabolic Rejectivity Syndrome" hypothesis. It became apparent that each individual may discover certain foods that, if eaten habitually, overstimulate the immune response of the body and cause a stressful malfunction of the immune system. The result is increased potential for chronic and degenerative disease.

This potential can also be diminished or reversed, even in the case of a chronic ailment of long duration. The Kaslow Medical Self-Care Program now offered in Santa Barbara, Newport Beach, and San Diego, California, has evolved from my accumulation of evidence. The program is based on teaching each patient self-care techniques in:

1. *Response Diet* testing of foods to identify foods rejected by the body.

2. Selection of a wholesome, balanced nutrition program excluding the rejected food.

3. Establishment of an individually workable exercise program to revitalize misused physical systems and improve oxygen (aerobic) conversion through *Stress/Stamina Balancing*.

4. Creation of an environment of care and support for the patient and family through *Dialogue in Human Concerns*, ensuring that everyone supports the assumption that the patient can and will improve.

5. Rebalancing the body's energy with *Response Point Therapy* (electroacupuncture).

These patient-education processes, designed to support the built-in self-regulating and self-healing systems of the body, have now superseded "usual and standard" treatments. We are cognizant of the effects; we try to uncover its cause and communicate it to the patient. The primary focus of our program is then to initiate support for the patient's self-healing systems. Essentially, all our patients experience a similar regime, regardless of the variety of their symptoms.

Of primary importance, we have seen that diseases written off as hopeless and incurable—multiple sclerosis, arthritis, diabetes, depression—may very well be the result of long-term food rejection and nutritional imbalance. When these and other stresses are removed, the person's system finds a way to restore its own balance. *The body knows best how to heal the disease!*

In this book, we offer simple and straightforward steps anyone can take to assist the rebalancing and revitalization of the body. The Kaslow Program points to new directions for those who seek a path beyond helplessness toward a more active and fulfilling life.

Arthur L. Kaslow, M.D.
Solvang, California

PART I

The
Kaslow Premise

1

SEEKING NEW PATHWAYS TO HEALTH

The real voyage of discovery consists not in seeking new landscapes, but in having new eyes; in seeing the universe with the eyes of another, or of a hundred others. And, in seeing the hundred universes each of them sees.

MARCEL PROUST

THERE ARE THREE IMPORTANT MESSAGES IN THIS BOOK for anyone experiencing a chronic and degenerative disease, or for anyone seeking continuing good health and well-being. Each message involves having new eyes, a fresh outlook. Only by seeing ourselves and our world differently than we have in the past can we find new pathways to health.

First, a previously unsuspected perspective of the role of nutrition in chronic disease is being discovered by many clinicians and researchers. At the Kaslow Medical Self-Care Center in Santa Barbara, California, we have learned that food allergy, more specifically *food rejectivity*, is a major factor in the development and persistence of degenerative disease. Balanced nutrition, which supplies the body with its needs for action energy, tissue building, and successful self-regulation, is essential, but it is not the complete story. In addition, each person must identify and remove from the diet those foods that the body cannot metabolize because of a persistent allergic response that has progressed to the body's complete rejection of these foods.

An individual's sensitivity to certain foods apparently builds up a rejectivity response over time. Specific foods unique to each person are rejected during digestion and metabolism, setting in motion a chain of events in the immune system that continues to weaken what is an already overstressed body.

Using a simple one-at-a-time Response Diet testing of foods, anyone can quickly determine those foods his or her system will not tolerate. *Removing those foods from the diet will stop the degenerative process of disease in most cases* and allow the body to set into motion its own natural healing process.

Second, we are seeing the amazing inner wisdom of the human body in a new light. Based on experiences with infectious diseases such as tuberculosis, smallpox, diphtheria, and malaria, we came to believe that *all* diseases were caused by invasion from outside. Experience at the Kaslow Center indicates that chronic and degenerative diseases (for example, arthritis, multiple sclerosis, cardiovascular disorders, diabetes) are more likely caused by long-term distortions of the body's built-in self-regulation systems.

Through this natural wisdom of self-regulation, each human body seeks balance and wellness. At the Kaslow Center we have designed our program around the major factors influencing this natural self-regulation. Through recognition of rejected foods, nutritional imbalances, emotional and psychological stresses, and limitations imposed by outdated cultural beliefs and attitudes about disease, we help design the program for each individual that can reverse the process of disease and dysfunction through personal choice and personal action.

Third, and perhaps most important, all of the factors that influence the course of chronic and degenerative diseases are simple, easy to understand, and *completely under the control of anyone willing to undertake a program of change for the better.*

Disease itself is complex. Doctors want to know all the many cellular and biochemical events that occur in the body so that medicine can manipulate these events to correct the symptoms.

Yet achieving health is simple. It involves supporting the natural self-regulating and self-healing systems of the body that *already know how to correct the disease.*

Therefore, the Kaslow Program is designed to educate the individual on how to build his or her own health and is not intended to treat a disease. There are no drugs and no expensive and prolonged treatments. Nor is there a continuing dependency on medical professionals who may deprive you of your sense of destiny and self-control. Instead, there are simple procedures you can learn to undertake by yourself. Your future is now in your hands. Many of the simple concepts and exercises in this book can show you how to achieve freedom from your pains and illnesses.

However, simple is not necessarily the same thing as easy. The concepts and ideas in this book are understandable and can be called "simple." But the actions they require may prove more difficult. The Kaslow Program is based on the notion that disease results when we make unwise choices that lead to a distortion of our natural self-regulation processes. To reverse these distortions, we must make new choices—in nutrition, stress situations, activity and exercise, and in attitudes about ourselves and disease. After years of habit, changing the way we make choices can be difficult. One of the primary goals of this book is to explain the alternatives and thus ease the discomfort of these changes. *What you decide to do is the primary determinant of the outcome.* No one but you can make your body well. After you have become familiar with the program and its concepts, Chapter 8, "A Personal Workbook for Health," offers a comprehensive set of ideas and exercises you can use to create your own plan for wellness.

PATIENTS FEEL DEPENDENT AND HELPLESS

By far the majority of people seeking care at the Kaslow Medical Self-Care Centers have been experiencing a significant physical disorder for an extended period of time. The shortest period is about 5 years; many have suffered for 10 or 15 years; some, for much longer. The typical case is one of gradual degeneration and loss of function through the years, resulting in the use of walkers, wheelchairs, or canes. Others may not experience difficulty in walking, but they tell of long-term pains, dysfunctions, and episodes of disability.

As we explore further in Chapter 6, "Moving from Helplessness to Action," the progression of events these patients unfold before us is almost always of dependency on their illness and the medical profession's definition of its possible future (or lack of one). This leads to feelings of hopelessness and inaction while the individual waits for science to find a magic cure for the dread disease. The patient is trapped by the assumed notion that nothing can be done until the medical profession designs a drug or course of action to "defeat" the disease. The long journey into this feeling of powerlessness is one of frustration and confusion.

Imagine yourself walking briskly across a room, engaged in your daily routine. Suddenly, as if the room had lurched to one side and caused you to lose your balance, you must reach for a chair, the wall, or a door frame. A concerned person nearby notices and asks if you are alright. You discover you cannot answer promptly. Your words are slurred. The coordination of your speech requires fierce concentration.

The first time this happens, you pass the event off as a brief occurrence of dizziness, perhaps a slight fever or fainting spell. You are shortly back in control. Walking and talking again become unconsciously routine. The second and third time this happens you become deeply frightened. "What's wrong with me? Am I losing my mind?"

Linda Dunlap was an energetic, active dispensary nurse for the Huntington Beach Police Department in mid-1974. She had seen many people brought into police custody intoxicated, emotionally upset, or otherwise unable to manage their physical actions. She knew how easy it was to assume someone had been taking drugs, drinking, or in some way overloading their body's capacity to maintain equilibrium.

This time *she* was the one losing her balance and her ability to speak clearly. She had taken no drugs, was not drunk, and had no other ready explanation for what was happening to her. Terrified, she had to find out what might be wrong.

On the advice of her physician, Linda entered the hospital for a five-day series of extensive tests. At first, it was thought that a hematoma (sac of fluid) had accumulated beneath her skull as a result of some overlooked bump on the head, exerting pressure on the brain and interfering with her functional motor control. There was concern that this sac might have burst. No hematoma was found.

Linda was released from the hospital with no clear diagnosis. She became increasingly concerned. She also became aware that anxiety and confusion were draining her of a great deal of energy. She would work a busy shift at the police department, come home, and drop into bed. If she quit working and had no continuing reason to move about, she feared that she might collapse and die. Linda felt compelled to go to work every day.

Linda lived one day at a time. She feared not knowing what was happening to her and how and when it might end. Most likely, according to her fears, her condition would continue to deteriorate.

She returned to her physician, pleading for more information about her problem. Because of her medical training and experience, she desired more concrete knowledge about why her body was failing. Reluctantly, her physician told her what he had apparently known for some time: Linda had multiple sclerosis.

Multiple sclerosis is the gradual deterioration of scattered patches of myelin sheath, a plastic wrap-like covering that surrounds the bundles of nerves throughout the nervous system. This covering is somewhat similar to the insulation on electric wires. When the continuity of the myelin sheath breaks down, the nerve signals travelling through the body become erratic. Information to the brain from sensors and muscles may be blocked or distorted and signals from the brain to the operational centers of the body may be misdirected or misinterpreted. Action coordination becomes confused. A routine task like lifting a leg or forming words requires extreme effort as the body's muscles must somehow figure out what the brain is telling them to do.

Since this activity within the body is normally almost totally automatic, loss of coordinated function is very frightening. The person feels out of control, helpless, confused, and frustrated. It is not uncommon for multiple sclerosis patients to become very angry at their bodies (looking at them as somehow separate entities) for being unable to perform what has been so routinely expected of them.

Linda experienced all of this frustration and helplessness. Then there was more news from her doctor: "Nothing can be done. Multiple sclerosis is considered incurable. Since we don't know what to do for your problem, it is best you go home and learn to live with it. It's useless for you to plan on coming back for more medical care. There is nothing I can really do to help you."

Now she was completely helpless and hopeless! At times, she felt panic-stricken. Faced with the terrifying experiences of her illness, never knowing when she would be unable to stand, walk, talk, or function effectively, Linda compromised as best she could with her life's responsibilities.

Her home life was completely disrupted. She spent most of the time in bed when she was not at work. Linda forced herself to continue her work, because she feared desperately what might happen to her if she gave up. It might be pointed out that by this time most people would have been in a wheelchair accepting and adjusting to the role of life-long invalid.

Linda's story up to this point is, unfortunately, all too typical. In Chapter 6 we elaborate on this feeling of helplessness created by the current medical approach to chronic and degenerative diseases. Linda, with her dynamic attitude, sought and found a way out of her seemingly hopeless situation.

DISCOVERING A NEW POSSIBILITY

One night Linda's mother telephoned, her voice filled with excitement. She had just seen a physician on television who related multiple sclerosis to specific nutritional problems of the individual patient. He was using a new nutritional approach to overcome the disease. His name was Dr. Arthur Kaslow, but in her excitement she had not heard where this doctor had his practice.

Linda had some difficulty locating Dr. Kaslow. She phoned the television network in New York. She phoned the national Multiple Sclerosis Society. She phoned the local station. No one seemed to know Dr. Kaslow's location or more about his work. Finally, she contacted the Arnold Pike Nutrition Show in Los Angeles and was informed that Dr. Kaslow had offices in Santa Barbara, California. Linda was relieved to learn that he was nearby, but remembering what her doctor had told her about multiple sclerosis, she was afraid to hope. The doctor might be of no help at all.

On December 15, 1975, Linda first visited the Kaslow Medical Self-Care Center in Santa Barbara. She was suspicious. The open atmosphere was unusual. This was not the indifferent, cold, and stiff professional environment she had known. One difference in particular caught her attention. She had previously been unable to get her physicians to share openly what was happening in her body. Dr. Kaslow said, without her asking, "By the time you leave here, you will know all we know about multiple sclerosis. You must understand and accept your disease in order to move on."

As Linda began the activities at the Kaslow Center, her feelings of helplessness began to wane. She found that her own actions affected her condition and that *she* could choose those actions that made her feel better.

She had given little thought to nutrition in relationship to her illness. Linda ate four or five chocolate bars and drank as much as a six-pack of cola drinks each day. Her diet was high in salt. She discovered that eating these foods caused an almost immediate return and worsening of her symptoms but that substituting other foods improved her condition.

Linda learned to plan her meals around wholesome, fresh foods. She chose more fresh vegetables, less fat, very little salt, and completely left out sugar, chocolate, and cola drinks. And, she found it was necessary to eliminate foods generally considered healthy from her diet—for example, wheat and dairy products—because she experienced varying degrees of difficulty after meals containing these foods.

While at the Kaslow Center, Linda learned about Response Point Therapy for tonification and revitalization of the body's natural self-regulation systems (see Chapter 7, "The Kaslow Medical Self-Care Program"). She was taught how to do a self-tonification treatment whenever she sensed weakness or oncoming symptoms and took home a small stimulator she could use for these treatments. Her muscle systems and nerve message systems in her body were reeducated through Stress/Stamina exercises learned at the Center. Skeptical at first, Linda decided to stay with it. So far, it was working beautifully; she had little to lose and much to gain.

Within a few months dramatic changes occurred. Linda regained control of her urinary bladder. Her feet, which had been weak and dragged when she walked, became functional again. She began to feel more assured physically and mentally competent as she moved through her day.

Her most important realization was that she was not a victim of multiple sclerosis. When problems appeared, she learned to find clues to their origin and to use new methods to deal with them and to avoid them in the future. She regained control of her life and discovered a new sense of self-confidence.

Linda still works part-time for the Huntington Beach Police Department, but she also has a new job. On her own initiative, she has opened a satellite office for Dr. Kaslow in Newport Beach, California. She spends three days a week there meeting with a growing number of people who arrive feeling, as she did four years ago, helpless and burdened by their diseases.

Two important patients were nearby. Her husband had suffered for some time with chronic headaches, her child with persistent bronchitis. At first, she thought it pointless to try the Kaslow Program for them because their problems were so different from her own. When she did go ahead, all were pleasantly surprised. The headaches and the bronchitis disappeared as all three members of the Dunlap family joined in a new awareness of their nutrition choices, life stresses, and the need for balance within the body.

Linda Dunlap is but one (or three if we include her family) of the many people who have successfully visited the Kaslow Medical Self-Care Centers for relief from chronic and degenerative diseases. Her patients in Newport Beach have a hard time believing she was ever disabled and helpless. Linda is now showing others the relatively simple and self-directed steps anyone can take to find freedom from disabling illness.

CLINICAL EXPERIENCE AND LABORATORY RESEARCH

Based on clinical experience with hundreds of patients who have learned the Kaslow Program and persisted in its application, we know that chronic and degenerative diseases can be reversed.

Yet, laboratory researchers tell us there are no "cures" for these problems.

For the sake of clarity, let's list the disorders that typify almost all the cases brought to the Kaslow Medical Self-Care Centers:

Alcoholism	Hypoglycemia
Arthritis	Intestinal disorders
Asthma	Listlessness and fatigue
Bronchitis	Migraine
Cardiovascular disorders	Multiple sclerosis
(heart diseases)	Neurosensory deafness
Colitis	Obesity
Depression	Psoriasis
Diabetes	Tinnitis
Digestive disorders	(ringing in the ears)
Eczema	Tobacco addiction
Hypertension	Traumatic injury

With the one exception of traumatic injury, all of these problems involve *systemic dysfunction*. By this we mean that some functional process in the body is failing, resulting in the symptoms we then name as a disease. In Chapter 2, "Where Is the Answer to Chronic Disease?" we explore more fully the direction traditional medical research has taken in its quest for answers to the causes and cures for disease. For now, let's look at a different approach—one we think accounts for the success of the Kaslow Program.

As we explain in detail later, traditional allopathic ("against pathology") medicine views disease as a natural enemy, invading the body from the outside. On the basis of this point of view, treatments involve drugs, surgery, or other interventions designed to manipulate or modify the symptoms—the visible effects— introduced by the invader. Hence, most research is directed toward identification of these invaders in order to combat them and their effects. Little research is directed toward investigating the life of the patient, nor to correlation of the appearance of symptoms with life events.

In addition to the allopathic view of attacking the visible effects of disease, there are two other approaches. One of these is to view disease as a failure of the natural self-healing and self-regulating systems within the body. An organism's tendency to return to a naturally balanced condition is called *homeostasis,* literally, "the same state." Any event experienced by the body will cause a corresponding response that tends to maintain system balance and function. We explain this concept more completely in Chapter 4, "The Amazing Process of Self-Regulation." Using this perspective of health and illness, a treatment program can be designed to rebalance and revitalize the self-regulation systems of the body so that the innate healing processes can proceed undisturbed.

Another view is to consider the emotional and physical context of the life situation of the person experiencing the disease. Practitioners looking from this perspective are interested in discovering those aspects of an individual's life that may affect general health and well-being. Nutritional habits, interpersonal-relationship stresses, work anxieties, money worries, concern about ill health, exercise patterns, changes in a home situation, and many other factors in a person's emotional life can affect general health. In addition, interaction with toxins in the environment, such as lead from gasoline, can have a significant effect on health.

These two perspectives are closely related; those factors in a person's life or environment that stress the body may become the cause of distortions in the body's systems of self-regulation. As an example, one might be able to handle a minimal exposure to lead or a few months' worry about money problems, but should these stresses persist for months or years without resolution they begin to distort the body's natural capacity to adapt to changes in the environment.

The Kaslow Medical Self-Care Program is designed to take these life-process aspects of disease into account rather than to seek the "one causative agent" stressed by traditional medical care. Dr. Kaslow is a clinical practitioner, not a research technician. We feel it is more important to find ways to improve the patient's general condition and at the same time prove what is causing the problem to the patient.

For example, in Linda Dunlap's case mentioned earlier, the patient's "treatment" began with a several years' search for an accurate diagnosis. The essence of this search was to isolate the entity (germ, virus, bacteria, or other agent) causing her symptoms. Using this single focus, it was believed that only when the agent was isolated could effective treatment begin. Unfortunately, *no specific causative agent has ever been isolated for multiple sclerosis.* Therefore, once the diagnosis had been verified, the physician was powerless to act because there was nothing to act against.

The patient, Linda, was left in a hopeless quandary: powerless to act, because the traditional medical system is based on the assumption that the patient is a passive receiver of professional instructions. It is presumed that there is nothing a patient can do on his/her own that would have any significant effect on a disease.

However, if one takes the view that disease can be ameliorated by rebalancing and revitalizing the body's self-healing processes and by exploring the factors in a person's life that may contribute to the decline of health, then efforts to reverse the disease and restore health can be made *without even knowing what the disease is,* or while the search for the diagnosis is proceeding. Using the Kaslow Medical Self-Care Program it is not difficult to support and preserve good health before disease symptoms ever appear.

In Linda's case, while she knew that she had multiple sclerosis and that traditional medicine had no remedy for her disease, the Kaslow Medical Self-Care Program offered her immediate steps she could take to rebalance and revitalize her body so that it could then *heal the disease by itself.* The body knows how to be well.

FIVE KEY BALANCING
AND VITALIZING FACTORS

If we suppose that the human body is a natural self-healing and self-regulating organism, then we must ask why does a person become susceptible to disease? Or one might ask, "If the body is self-healing, why does *anyone* become ill?" Our clinical experience at the Kaslow Centers has led to an investigation of these key factors that might influence or distort the body's self-regulation. We knew that if we could identify these factors and patients could take action to alleviate their impact on the body, people experiencing disease could get well, regardless of the source of the disease. We have found five key elements that appear to set off the gradual deterioration that is the earmark of chronic disease.

Metabolic Rejectivity

Our clinical experience indicates that most people experiencing chronic physical or mental problems habitually eat foods that their bodies cannot assimilate or metabolize. These foods, normally considered nutritious and beneficial, are rejected by the body each time they are eaten, overloading the immune system and distorting self-regulation. This results ultimately in the failure of important maintenance processes in the various body organs, such as heart, lungs, nervous system and muscles. These rejected foods are unique to each individual. There are no standard formulas which can produce a miracle diet for any specific disease occurring in different patients. This syndrome is explained more completely in Chapter 3, "The Metabolic Rejectivity Syndrome (MRS): A Working Hypothesis."

Through one-at-a-time food testing, as described in Chapter 8, any individual can discover those foods he or she rejects and eliminate them from the diet. As a result, the immune system is not overstimulated and the body gains an opportunity to restore damaged organs to an effective functional state.

Nutritional Imbalance

As we detail in Chapter 5, "Good Food, Vitamins, and Minerals," Americans have developed food habits that do not support health and well-being. In addition to identifying non-tolerated foods, each person must learn to establish a nutritious diet that will supply all the body's needs for action energy, tissue maintenance, and continuing self-regulation. In *Nutrition Counseling* at the Kaslow Centers and in the workbook in Chapter 8, simple concepts are offered to lead the way to a healthy diet.

Unresolved Stress

In Chapter 4, "The Amazing Process of Self-Regulation," we describe how the accumulated effect of significant events in one's life ("Piling It On") or a continuing unresolved conflict (the "Double Bind") can cause a chronic distortion of many of the body's routine maintenance processes. Over time, this leads to pain, failure of organ function, and disease. In the Kaslow Program's *Dialogue in Human Concerns* and in several of the exercises in the Chapter 8 workbook, we teach the skills needed to identify and effectively relax emotional stress.

Lack of Movement/Lack of Oxygen

Our convenience-oriented sedentary lifestyle limits the activity of the body. People experiencing serious illness become even more inactive than usual. As discussed throughout the book, the body needs movement and oxygen to function at the level of wellness. Without continuing movement, which stimulates the heart/lung system, gradual decline of the body results from lack of adequate oxygen utilization.

The Stress/Stamina Balancing program, described in Chapter 7, "The Kaslow Medical Self-Care Program," is designed to promote body flexibility and oxygen-conversion capacity. A section of the Chapter 8 workbook is devoted to exercises you can learn to do at home. A by-product of the development of flexibility and stamina in the body is an improved capacity to deal with physical and emotional stress—thus the name "Stress/Stamina."

A Helpless or Powerless Attitude

By far the most important obstacle to overcome for those experiencing serious or chronic illness is the idea that they have no power to change the situation. As we explore in Chapter 6, this feeling of helplessness stems from the current medical view of disease which places all power in the hands of the professional. If you quickly review the factors we have listed here, you will see that they are all dependent on processes built into the habits and choices of an individual. Therefore, they all *can be changed* once you start thinking "wellness" rather than "illness."

The personnel at the Kaslow Centers aid each patient by reinforcing the notion that he or she can and will get better as a result of new choices, which the patient can easily learn to make. This assumption, plus the Dialogue in Human Concerns, offers the incentive and inspiration to change. There are several ideas in Chapter 8 to help clarify your views on your power to affect change in your life.

Another feature of the Kaslow Program is directed specifically at rebalancing systems within the body. Response Point Therapy, as described in Chapter 7, employs a unique adaptation of ancient Chinese acupuncture to reestablish the flow of energies throughout the body.

A COMPARISON OF VIEWS

Throughout this chapter we have introduced a number of new concepts about disease that are amplified later in the book. Because the Kaslow Program is based on assumptions quite different from those of traditional medicine, let's clarify these differences by a comparative review:

ASSUMPTIONS OF TRADITIONAL ALLOPATHIC MEDICINE	ASSUMPTIONS OF THE KASLOW MEDICAL SELF-CARE PROGRAM
1. Nature makes many mistakes. Through scientific manipulation, we can fix these errors.	1. Nature is wise. In our lack of wisdom we make mistakes, but through education we can learn to avoid them.
2. Chronic disease (and all disease) is caused by the invasion of the body by outside agents. The invasion is generally beyond human control unless effective immunizations can be developed or the agents eliminated.	2. Chronic disease is caused by the failure of natural self-healing (homeostatic) systems within the body. This failure is the result of unwise life choices made due to a lack of proper awareness.
3. The key to alleviation of chronic disease is the elimination of, or control	3. The key to alleviation of a chronic disease is the rebalancing and

Against Disease

ASSUMPTIONS OF TRADITIONAL ALLOPATHIC MEDICINE	ASSUMPTIONS OF THE KASLOW MEDICAL SELF-CARE PROGRAM
of, the symptoms of the disease.	revitalization of the distorted homeostatic processes of the body.
4. The purpose of diagnosis is to identify an entity that has attacked the body, causing the disease.	4. The purpose of diagnosis is to identify those life processes that lead to distortion of the natural self-regulation systems within the body.
5. The purpose of treatment is to modify or remove the symptoms of a disease.	5. The purpose of treatment is to educate the patient, rebalance the self-regulation systems, and establish new habits that will stop the distortion of these self-regulation processes.
6. Drugs are used, as is surgery, to manipulate the natural structure of the body to eliminate, suppress, or modify symptoms.	6. Drugs and surgery are avoided as much as possible. They are seen as stressors that further distort self-regulation.
7. Patients expect a quick response to drug and surgical therapies for chronic problems. This is based on previous experience with infectious disease.	7. Patients realize that a process that took years to develop may take some time to reverse.
8. The focus of concern is disease, disability, and limitations. "Side effects" from drugs and surgery are acceptable risks.	8. The focus is on healthy function, lifestyle, and positive alternatives. There are no undesirable side effects.

ASSUMPTIONS OF TRADITIONAL ALLOPATHIC MEDICINE	ASSUMPTIONS OF THE KASLOW MEDICAL SELF-CARE PROGRAM
9. Responsibility for outcome is controlled by the physician.	9. Responsibility for outcome is controlled by the patient.
10. The patient is dependent on professional authority and experiences feelings of personal incompetence and loss of control. Failure is judged to be patient incompetence rather than professional inadequacy.	10. The patient is buoyed up by knowledgeable support, caring, and the belief that he or she can and will get well as a result of personal action.

THE ELEMENTS OF SUCCESS

Hundreds of patients have visited the Kaslow Center in Santa Barbara, California. Many have succeeded in channeling their illness and life in new directions of promise and well-being. A review of many cases and interviews with a number of patients gave us some insights into those who succeed.

Motivation to find a way out.   Many patients have succeeded in overcoming their illnesses in the face of medical advice that they were wasting their time and money in attempting to change what was. These patients refused to accept the sentence that "nothing could be done" for many chronic diseases. Many felt an intuitive resistance to drugs and surgery. Others had undergone extensive treatment with little improvement. Those who maintained their motivation to get well and came to us were those people who felt they must retain a measure of control over their destiny.

A willingness to accept the disease as something they could do something about.   These patients refused to take the "victim" position our society asks us to assume when disease occurs. Although many patients have been angered and frustrated by their

disorders, the ones who succeed with our program do not per-
ceive their disease as an enemy to be crushed or killed.

Interest in self-knowledge.   Successful patients want to know
more about their bodies and how they work. Because they do
not see their disease as an enemy from "without," they realize
they can work with the processes of the body to regain control
of their lives and their activities.

Sensitivity to their own body processes.   Successful patients
report a keener awareness of the stresses in their lives, responses
to eating habits, and knowledge of factors that cause discomfort.
They become more sensitive to the need to change personal
habits, diet, or exercise routines to meet new circumstances.
They are wary of the formula diet or exercise program and have
learned to respect and understand their individuality.

Persistence in carrying out a self-designed program.   Everyone we know who has persisted in the Kaslow Program has
improved. Many patients achieve remarkable success while visiting the Kaslow Center only to experience a setback when they
return to their routine in the home environment. This difficulty
may be attributable to lack of support from family, friends, or
health care professionals who do not recognize the possibility
that the patient can and will improve. Without this support,
old habits and nutritional patterns may reemerge and problems
may return. Those who adhere to the program and establish a
support system of family and friends or maintain their personal
fortitude continue to improve.

The purpose of this book is to describe what happens at the
Kaslow Self-Care Centers, to show you the steps you can take
toward a better understanding of any chronic problems with
your body, and to explore why this fairly simple method is not
more widely practiced. There are no amazing drugs or miracle
treatments available at the Kaslow Self-Care Centers. The Kaslow
Program is the result of a different perspective of the nature of
chronic disease and the acceptance of the premise that *the body
knows how to heal itself.*

2

WHERE IS THE ANSWER TO CHRONIC DISEASE?

WHO IS THE "VICTIM" OF A HEART ATTACK—THE HEART or the person in whom the heart beats? Who is the attack*er* and who the attack*ee*? When someone experiences an "attack" of arthritis, bursitis, upset stomach, muscle spasm, or tennis elbow, what (or who) is doing the attacking?

In a booklet distributed by the Muscular Dystrophy Association of America, the deeply touching story of Richard Kisonak includes this language: "A mysterious, fatal disease . . . has quietly and determinedly been *waging a hellish war* on my muscular system." Later in this same brochure, Dr. Jacob A. Brody says, "*Victims* are usually *stricken* in the prime of life" [emphasis added].

This language, which most accept almost without question in this society, strengthens the assumption of an *adversary relationship* between a disease and the person experiencing the disease. Society teaches us to "declare war," whether on inflation, depression, big business, air pollution, crime, or disease. Any aspect of the culture which is out of order can be found described by the media as an *enemy* to be fought, conquered, or killed. Persons experiencing the effects of these phenomena are cast as powerless *victims*. This powerless-victim position is, unfortunately, held by almost everyone experiencing a chronic, degenerative disease.

The question foremost in a patient's mind when he or she seeks care from a physician is most frequently "What can you do for me?" With only a few exceptions, patients arriving at the Kaslow Medical Self-Care Centers come with this question in their minds. A fairly typical dialogue might be:

PATIENT:

I have been to see so many doctors and tried so many treatments. Nothing seems to work, and I am getting worse instead of better. I've heard about your program, Dr. Kaslow, and I've come hoping you can help me. Can you make me well again? [The patient's words may not be that explicit, but the message is usually clear and the tone pleading.]

DR. KASLOW:

I doubt if I can "make you well again." That is beyond my power to do. However, if you have a sincere desire to become well and are able and willing to review some of the factors in your life that aggravate your condition and change them, then most likely you can and will improve.

The patient's perspective is usually such that he/she thinks that he/she is a helpless victim of disease and is totally dependent on medical science to fight the battle against the disease and *fix* the problem. Dr. Kaslow's perspective, as we have discussed before, is that the body is a natural self-healing system and the factors disturbing this system must be recognized and modified. The patient has recognized little of the relationship between nutrition, attitudes, life habits, and disease. To Dr. Kaslow, these are the central issues in ameliorating or curing a disease.

THE NEED TO BE MADE WELL

Historically, there have been two distinct positions taken in regard to disease and health: (1) when disease occurs, we are essentially ill and must be *made well* through the services of a professional healer; or (2) we are essentially healthy and well and must be *made ill* for disease to occur. We quote Thomas McKeown from *The Modern Rise of Population*:

> In the classical tradition there are two ideas concerning man's health:
>
>> One, associated with the goddess Hygeia, that health could be achieved by a rational way of life; the other, personified by the god Aesculapius, that health depended largely on the role of the physician as the healer of the sick.
>
> Both concepts are found in the Hippocratic writings and they have survived in medical thought and practice down to the present day. However, since the 17th Century at least, the Aesculapian approach has been dominant. Philosophically, it derived support from Descartes' concept of the living organism as a machine which might be taken apart and reassembled if its structure and function were understood. Practically, it seemed to find confirmation in the work of Kepler and Harvey and in the success of the physical sciences in manipulating inanimate matter. It is only in the past few decades that it has become evident that his interpretation is quite inaccurate, that the health of man is determined essentially by his behavior, his food, and the nature of the world around him, and is only marginally influenced by personal medical care. We have been taught to believe that *we are ill and are made well*; it is nearer the truth to say that *we are well and are made ill*.

NATURE AS AN ADVERSARY

Western technological and scientific progress rests on certain Judeo-Christian/Greek assumptions about humanity and the world. The book of *Genesis* tells us that because of our knowledge of good and evil, we are cursed and must work to overcome the inevitable ravages of nature if we are to regain the favor of God. This doctrine, placing humanity in a "one-down" position before a potentially angry God, was blended with Greek thought to produce a view of the world as full of dualities and conflict. We see ourselves as separate from nature, in contest both with nature and each other in a continuing battle for survival.

Joseph Chilton Pearce, in *Exploring the Crack in the Cosmic Egg*, notes, "Consider one of the basic assumptions of Western rational scientism: The life force on our planet has evolved one of its most magnificent expressions, the human mind, the function of which is supposedly to outwit and dominate the life force from which it evolved."

This adversary assumption, when applied through technology, encourages strategies designed to manipulate and control nature. As a result, rational thought and objective observation have produced an ever-growing body of knowledge about the particulars of physical phenomena but have failed to develop any understanding of the purpose and fulfillment of life. Robert Pirsig, in *Zen and the Art of Motorcycle Maintenance*, points out:

> The Greek Mythos has endowed our culture with the tendency underlying all the evil of our technology, the tendency to do what is reasonable even when it isn't any good. Reason and quality have become separated and in conflict with one another. Quality has been forced under and reason made supreme.

It is difficult, if not impossible, to find peace and fulfillment in an environment perceived as a constant or potential adversary.

Disease as a Weapon of Nature

Seeing nature as an adversary, it is not a big step to the Western view of disease as a weapon of nature intended to strike us down. A brief look at any newspaper or magazine discussing illness will quickly illustrate how our society views people experiencing disease as unwitting victims of a natural circumstance. As discussed earlier, if someone has a heart attack, or is stricken with arthritis, where is the attacker and who is doing the striking? We have thought of the attacker and striker as some malevolent force in nature that science must somehow conquer.

We discussed in Chapter 1 Linda Dunlap's long search for an answer to her undefined illness. During that search, she recalls feelings of being punished for some wrongdoing. Many patients express the question, "Why me?" This question implies that some universal force has chosen the patient as a victim. Such an assumption creates a sense of complete helplessness in what seems to be the face of powerful natural forces well beyond individual control. In such an adversary situation there must be an identifiable enemy. Because a direct confrontation with God is more than most of us have wanted to undertake, science has attempted to discover something more tangible and reachable.

Not much more than one hundred years ago, science's understanding of the nature of infections and antiseptics was just beginning. It was not understood why so many persons died of infections in hospitals. In 1846, when Ignaz Semmelweiss of Vienna noted an exceptionally high rate of death among patients whose doctors had recently performed autopsies, he initiated rules requiring doctors and workers to wash thoroughly between surgeries or autopsies. The death rate in his section of the hospital dropped significantly.

The implication, of course, was that human misunderstanding had caused the deaths, rather than natural actions. Although this may seem obvious to us now, and we would not necessarily *blame* the unwitting doctors for this lack of knowledge, this simple concept was not so graciously received by Dr. Semmelweiss's colleagues. The medical society rejected him and he was dismissed from the hospital. To assume that scientific strategies might have been responsible for disease and death was *heresy*. Even though medical science has changed in remarkable ways since the mid-1800s, this steadfast belief in nature as adversary and science as savior hangs on.

We have looked at disease as an enemy and have sought through science and human ingenuity to locate the enemy and declare war. To assume that our own actions might be contributing to the problem has been made unthinkable.

The Enemy Revealed

Robert Margotta reports in *The Story of Medicine*:

Increasing awareness of the nature of contagion led to a search for the agents which actually caused the diseases. The microscope, which had now been brought to an advanced state of development, allowed close study of the appearance of tissues in health and disease. Knowledge of the structure and function of the body *at the cellular level* progressed rapidly. The greatest name in pathology was Rudolph Virchow, who systematized the subject and stated that diseases were manifested in the cells [emphasis added].

In 1858, Virchow reported that "disease is nothing but the reactions of the cells to the causative agent of the disease." The search for specific enemies was on. The notion that nature had created a host of adversaries to make our lives miserable was validated. Between 1850 and 1910:

- Pasteur discovered that the organisms that caused putrefaction in wine and milk could be killed by heating the substance.

- Pasteur discovered the anthrax bacilli and devised an inoculation to prevent anthrax in farm animals.

- Pasteur isolated the rabies virus and devised a rabies vaccination.

- Pierre Roux and G.A.E. Yersin isolated the diphtheria bacillus; Yersin the bubonic plague bacillus.

- Robert Koch isolated the tubercle bacillus.

- Patrick Manson discovered the parasite carried by a mosquito that transmits elephantiasis.

- Carlos Finlay identified the mosquito that carries yellow fever.

- Charles Alphonse found the cause of malaria—a parasite carried by mosquitos.

- Charles Nicolle found the louse that transmits typhus fever.

The parade of enemies continued to be identified, and a growing rogues' gallery was made available for the microscopic sleuth. However, it was another 50 years before the effective instruments of battle were made available in the war against infectious diseases. In 1935, Gerhard Domagk introduced sulfanilamide, the first chemical antibiotic. Alexander Fleming, Howard

Florey, and Ernst Chain introduced penicillin in 1940, and Schatz, Bugie, and Waksman followed with streptomycin in 1944. The effectiveness of these drugs was proven in World War II, minimizing infections from wounds and field surgery and reducing the effects of exposure to diseases not native to the home environment of the far-ranging soldiers. Medicine now had "medical bullets" it could shoot at disease targets resulting from bacterial infections.

DISEASE PATTERNS CHANGE

Figure 2.1 shows us that although our identification and control of infectious diseases have become more successful, a new set of problems has emerged to take their place: chronic, degenerative diseases. Whereas acute, infectious diseases accounted for almost 700 deaths per 100,000 population in 1900, they now account for fewer than 20. In 1900, chronic disease accounted for fewer than 400 deaths per 100,000 population; in 1970, more than 700. (The spike to about 900 deaths per 100,000 population for infectious diseases in the 1917-1919 period represents an influenza epidemic during those years.) Glazier predicts that of every 100 males now born in the United States, 83 are likely to suffer and eventually die of a chronic disease.

Table 2.1 lists the ten most prevalent causes of death in the United States both in 1900 and 1970.

Note that tuberculosis, gastroenteritis (intestinal inflammations), nephritis (kidney inflammations) and diphtheria have disappeared from the 1970 list. The death rates for influenza and pneumonia have been reduced to 15% of their earlier incidence. The illnesses catalogued here are all infectious diseases.

The *total* death rate per 100,000 dropped about 25% in 70 years; however, of the 832 deaths per one hundred thousand in 1970, 640 (80%) were caused by heart disease, cerebrovascular lesions, and cancer—all chronic diseases. Infectious disease, if it is an enemy, is retreating from the war. New to the 1970 list are diabetes, cirrhosis of the liver, and chronic respiratory problems— all of which are systemic malfunctions of the body rather than invasions of infectious agents.

Figure 2.1:   COMPARISON OF DEATHS
PER 100,000 POPULATION, 1900–1970

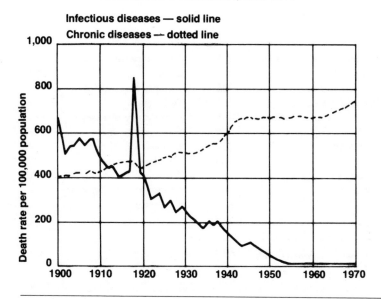

From "Task of Medicine," by William Glazier, *Scientific American*, Vol. 228, April 1973, pp. 13–17.

Death rates from heart disease and cancer have risen more than 250% since 1900. But these rates tell only part of the story. Infectious diseases usually appear rapidly and have fairly short and measurable lifespans. They are generally cured, heal naturally, or result in death within a relatively short time. Chronic diseases, on the other hand, appear slowly, cause gradual dysfunction or disability, persist after protracted treatments, and cause continuing hardship, both in terms of personal suffering and cost of treatment and care.

We see in Tables 2.2 and 2.3, excerpted from the *Historical Abstracts of the United States*, that during the time that deaths from infectious diseases have fallen and deaths from chronic disease have risen, *private and public expenditures for health care have grown logarithmically in the past 40 years.*

Research expenditures have grown from about $8 million in 1935 to $2.5 *billion* in 1975. Both personal and governmental

Table 2.1:   MOST PREVALENT CAUSES
OF DEATH IN THE UNITED STATES

1900		1970	
CAUSE	DEATHS/ 100,000	CAUSE	DEATHS/ 100,000
Influenza & pneumonia	201	Heart disease	360
Tuberculosis	198	Cancer	175
Gastroenteritis	145	Cerebrovascular lesions	105
Heart disease	135	Accidents	54
Cerebrovascular lesions	105	Circulatory diseases	31
Chronic nephritis	80	Influenza & pneumonia	30
Accidents	72	Diseases of infancy	21
Cancer	63	Diabetes mellitus	18
Diseases of infancy	62	Cirrhosis of the liver	15
Diphtheria	40	Bronchitis, emphysema, asthma	13
	1,101		832

From *Historical Abstracts of the United States*

expenditures for health care services have grown from about $7.5 billion in 1935 to more than $210 billion in 1975 and now account for more than 8% of all goods and services sold in the United States. In President Carter's State of the Union address in January 1979, he identified rising medical costs as one of our most serious national issues. Carter pointed out that medical costs are rising $1 million a day and doubling every five years.

Somehow this massive expenditure of money and effort is missing the mark. We are not finding the answers to our health care questions. The shift of greatest incidence from infectious disease, on which our current model of medical treatment is based, to chronic disease has not been properly acknowledged in our research and care delivery. The growing number of patients coming to the Kaslow Centers and the growing number of other "alternative" clinics and centers springing up around the country suggest that the traditional medical approach to chronic disease needs reevaluation.

Meanwhile, the war against chronic disease continues unabated. Even though chronic disease is very different in its mani-

Table 2.2:   U.S. HEALTH CARE EXPENDITURES

| | EXPENDITURES IN *MILLIONS* OF DOLLARS | |
	1935	1975
Total National Health	4,000	150,000
Personal Health Care	3,500	50,000
Retail Drug Sales	1,000	20,000
Medical Facilities Construction	60	4,000
Medical Research	8	2,500
	8,568	226,500

From *Historical Abstracts of the United States*

festations and causes from infectious disease, the traditional medical view of disease as an enemy to be identified and killed persists. Table 2.3 illustrates the magnitude of the effort of publicly supported agencies which wage this war.

Among these organizations alone, which do not include government and university research of perhaps an even greater magnitude, almost $70 million is spent each year searching for the answers to chronic diseases. Almost all this research is directed toward laboratory analysis of discrete cellular events in laboratory animals or humans. Almost none of the research explores life habits of individuals as these habits might affect disease or the involvement of systemic malfunction in the body. The underlying assumption about treatment by most of these research efforts is based on experience with the polio syndrome: A miracle breakthrough is anticipated. A causative germ or agent will be found, a miracle drug will be developed to kill the germ, and the disease will disappear—just as polio did after the discovery of the Salk and Sabin vaccines.

In the meantime, sufferers of these diseases are put "on hold" and told they can do nothing until science solves the riddle to their disease. However, this entire effort, growing consistently and at great expense since World War II, *has had little or no effect on the incidence of chronic disease in the United States!*

Table 2.3: PUBLICLY SUBSCRIBED CAMPAIGNS
TO CONQUER CHRONIC DISEASE

ORGANIZATION	FOUNDING DATE	RESEARCH DOLLARS LATEST YEAR	RESEARCH DOLLARS SINCE FOUNDING	NO. OF PEOPLE EXPERIENCING DISEASE, LATEST AVAILABLE YEAR
American Heart Association	1912	$214,260 (1977)	$310 million	40 million
American Cancer Society	1913	$44 million (1978)	$454 million	1+ million
Muscular Dystrophy Association	1950	$15 million (1977)	Not available	Not available
Multiple Sclerosis Society	1946	$3 million (1978)	$43 million	500,000
Arthritis Foundation	1948	$3.6 million (1977)	Not available	31 million
American Diabetes Association	1940	$1.8 million (1978)	$15 million since 1970	44 million (approx.)

From *Historical Abstracts of the United States*

More people are suffering from these diseases each year and science seems no closer to "winning the war" against them than it was 25 years ago.

The view that disease is a natural enemy, caused by the invasion of the body by germs, bacilli, viruses, and the like, and the laborious search through the microscope for the identity of these enemies at the cellular level of the body may so seriously limit the outlook on the problem that science will never find the answer for chronic, degenerative disease.

There is an ancient Sufi (Islamic) story about a man searching for something in front of his home. A friend happens by and offers assistance.

"Are you looking for something?"

"Yes, the key to my house."

"I will help you search."

The two combed the area for some time. The friend finally asked, "Where did you last see your key?"

"In my bedroom."

"Why, then, are we searching out here?"

"There is more light out here."

Although there may be light and interesting phenomena at the small end of the microscope, the answer to chronic, degenerative disease may not be found there. It may very well be that none of these diseases is the result of an invading entity. Therefore, to seek that entity so that we may attack it may never prove fruitful. An attack on the symptoms that signal a disease may prove to be an attack on some basic function of the body, further stressing an already weakened system.

Present Treatments May Be
Adding to the Problem

We are reminded of the story of Dr. Semmelweiss and his simple observation of the relationship between cleanliness and infection. Medicine would not believe that its methods of solving a problem were contributing to the problem. We may be in a very similar position now in regard to chronic, degenerative diseases.

Doctors, closed in by their view of disease as an attacking entity from nature, have great difficulty seeing the fairly simple relationship between nutrition, food allergy, lack of exercise, stress experience, and personal attitudes and chronic degenerative disease. They cannot imagine that if someone revitalizes the natural self-regulation processes of the body by redirecting nutritional choices, alleviating stress, and changing attitudes, the body will heal itself. Another barrier in the physicians' realization of this alternative view of chronic disease is the fact that the professional role of savior and rescuer disappears with this understanding of the problem. People do not need incredible technology, expensive diagnostic procedures, protracted treatments, and costly drugs. All they need to do is to rid themselves of the attitude of helplessness and professional dependency, to take action on their own to establish more productive nutritional, exercise, and stress management habits, and they will get better!

THE NEW ANSWER TO CHRONIC DISEASE

The Kaslow Medical Self-Care Program, as noted at the end of Chapter 1, assumes that chronic disease is not caused by invading entities but is the result of long-term distortion of natural self-regulation systems in the body. These systems have malfunctioned because of habitual life choices made by the persons experiencing the disease. We say this not *to blame* them for making such choices or to induce guilt. Had they known the consequences of the choices, they no doubt would not have made them. Our general ignorance of how our bodies work, our dependence on medical professionals to maintain our health, and our lack of attention to basic practices that maintain good health have all contributed to the problem.

In Chapter 6, "Moving from Helplessness to Action," we explore further this new perspective of chronic disease and how individuals can get beyond traditional attitudes to improved health. We assume that nature is wise—a friend rather than an enemy. As we have said before, the body essentially knows how to heal itself. Chronic disease can be *reversed*, and significant results can be achieved through personal actions (as explained in Chapter 8). It is not so much a matter of what Dr. Kaslow or this book can do for you, but what you are willing to do for yourself. It is a matter of self-knowledge and education.

Your body knows how to heal itself if you will give it nourishment and support. Treat it like a close friend. Help it and it will help you. Your body and disease are not enemies to be conquered.

Let us reiterate here some of the assumptions on which the Kaslow Program is based:

1. Chronic disease is the result of failure of the natural self-healing (homeostatic) systems of the body. This failure

is caused by poor life choices made through ignorance of the body's needs.

2. The key to the alleviation of chronic disease is the restoration of proper function of distorted self-regulation systems.

3. The purpose of diagnosis and evaluation is to identify those life factors that are distorting the self-regulation systems. These factors are: metabolic food rejection, nutritional imbalance, unresolved stress, inadequate oxygen for body maintenance (lack of exercise), attitudes concerning the disease, and one's power to affect the future.

4. The purpose of treatment and education is to establish a rebalance and revitalization of the body so that the inner wisdom of the body can return it to health.

The Kaslow Program does not treat the disease but restores the body's natural ability to maintain its own health. The key to the success of that process is within the person experiencing the disease. Hope, willingness to change, growing self-knowledge, and new sensitivities to stressful factors in life can change the world for a sufferer of chronic disease. After changing an individual's attitudes, the program removes from the person's diet those foods the body cannot tolerate, and supports the person's system with balanced nutrition and healthful exercise, resulting in new life horizons.

3

THE METABOLIC REJECTIVITY SYNDROME (MRS): A WORKING HYPOTHESIS

The mind and the diet relate to each other in a sort of double feedback fashion. What goes on psychologically affects how and what we eat in many ways. The resulting change in nutritional status has important effects in psychological and physical functioning. This means that a continuous interplay exists, and that this can, if allowed to run amok, carry one to great heights (or depths) of mental and physical disorder. Of course, with the proper understanding this interaction becomes the means of promoting the health of the whole person.

RUDOLPH BALLENTINE, M.D.,
Diet & Nutrition

DIANE M., A MULTIPLE SCLEROSIS PATIENT AT THE KAS-low Center, found that shortly after eating beefsteak her legs would not function. She needed a taxi to go just one block for a scheduled blood test. The following day, after eating a baked potato, her body seemed energized and she was able to walk easily along the same distance to the laboratory for another appointment.

Bonnie S., who weighed 262 pounds, was experiencing nausea, headaches, and fatigue. She found that when she ate eggs, cheese, asparagus, or wheat, she would experience severe bouts of rheumatoid arthritis in addition to her general feelings of malaise. If she walked a block, she needed to rest afterward for more than two hours. When she eliminated these foods from her diet, she lost 120 pounds in 8 months and now walks more than two miles each day.

A 16-year-old girl is apparently doomed to a lifetime of schizophrenia. After a four-day fast, she appears to be functioning normally. Given a glass of milk, she is psychotic within an hour.

A 32-year-old clergyman suffers from severe arthritis. After a brief fast, the symptoms disappear. Test meals of cane sugar and corn cause his joints to swell again.

The first two cases are drawn from clinical experience at the Kaslow Medical Self-Care Centers. The latter two are excerpted from *Dr. Mandell's 5-Day Allergy Relief System*, a new book by Marshall Mandell, M.D., and L. W. Scanlon. In each case, we saw an immediate physical response to the eating of certain foods. These responses are allergic or rejection responses. They produce effects that have been labeled as a specific disease with special symptoms.

THE BODY RESPONDS TO FOODS

Diane and Bonnie, the Kaslow patients, and the teenage girl and clergyman, Dr. Mandell's patients, discovered strong negative reactions to specific foods that seriously disrupted their normal body functions. Eating foods usually considered to be nutritionally beneficial, each experienced an internal response identified as "disease."

Until they had undertaken testing, *none of these people had ever associated eating habits with episodes of disease.* Once the issue was clearly raised, the connection seemed quite obvious. Here we have four chronic conditions—multiple sclerosis, obesity, schizophrenia, arthritis—all directly related by the experience of the patient to recurrent episodes of symptoms which followed meals of certain foods. And, these foods—beef, eggs, cheese, asparagus, wheat, milk, and corn—have never been considered potentially harmful to humans and are, in fact, looked to as sources of essential nutrients. Sugar, the other food listed, is a separate matter. Later in this chapter and in Chapter 5, we discuss further the role sugar appears to play in the onset and continuation of chronic and degenerative disorders.

Significantly, when these foods were no longer eaten, or when the person fasted, there was fairly immediate and dramatic improvement. The symptoms of the diagnosed disease either diminished or disappeared. Omitting these foods from the diet apparently gave the body an opportunity to reestablish its natural balance and set self-healing processes in motion. Once the stress of the foods each person's body could not tolerate was removed, improvement began.

Dr. Kaslow (California), Dr. Mandell (Connecticut), Dr. Theron Randolph (Illinois), and Dr. William Philpott (Oklahoma) are four physicians among a growing number across the country who are recognizing the critical role unusual responses to foods can play in chronic and degenerative disorders. The beauty of this concept is that it opens a new line of inquiry into chronic disorders and shows that they are easily *reversible.* The apparent conclusion is that these disorders result from long-term habits of eating foods the body cannot accept. The body's response to the foods sets into motion a chain of events leading to distortion of the self-regulation systems built in by nature. When the stress of these foods is removed, these self-regulation systems reestablish functional maintenance of the body, and the disease disappears (see Chapter 4, "The Amazing Process of Self-Regulation").

Another advantage of this concept is its *simplicity.* Through one-at-a-time Response Diet testing of foods, anyone can learn to identify the specific foods causing the problems and can then eliminate these foods from the diet. This requires no expensive medical treatment nor professional dependency (see Chapter 7 and Chapter 8). It illustrates that the body is designed to be healthy and simply needs to have stresses reduced in order to function properly.

Based on our clinical experience at the Kaslow Centers, we have developed a working hypothesis for the body process that leads to chronic and degenerative disorder through food rejection. This process seems to involve two related activities as the body digests, assimilates, and metabolizes foods: (1) gradual and cumulative distortion in the utilization of foods, especially carbohydrates, and (2) increasing involvement of the body's immune system as certain foods are "rejected."

MEASURING BODY RESPONSES

As an important phase of the Kaslow program, a group of patients gather each Tuesday morning for an unusual meal. Seated together in the reception area, each patient consumes approximately 103 grams of natural carbohydrate consisting of three oranges, six dates, and one banana. (A similar test is the glucose tolerance test, during which responses to sugar or sucrose are measured. We use real foods that contain fructose, the natural fruit sugar, in order to gain a more accurate picture of the individual's responses to *foods* as opposed to chemicals.)

One would normally not eat 103 grams of fruit at one sitting. The purpose of this overdose of fruit is twofold: (1) to gain some laboratory information concerning the individual's capacity to metabolize these foods, and (2) to give the individual a direct personal experience of the body's response to these foods.

Before eating the fruit and for 6½ hours afterward, several factors will be monitored to assess the person's reaction to this meal of fruit. Central to our discussion are the levels of glucose (blood sugar) checked hourly and the percentage of certain white blood cells, called *lymphocytes,* in the blood stream at 3½ and 6½ hours. These lymphocytes, as we explain more fully later, are the messengers and scavengers used by the total body's immune system to remove unwanted material from the body.

One lesson becomes increasingly apparent to each patient as the person keeps a diary during the day of the test: *What you eat affects how you feel.* At different times throughout the day,

many patients experience a myriad of psychological states, ranging from euphoria to extreme depression, and physical states,
ranging from hyperactivity to extreme fatigue and disability.
Most important, *many patients experience in an acute, intense
form the symptoms of the disease that brought them to the Center
for treatment.* Pains, dysfunctions, and disabilities, which are
at the core of their need for treatment, escalate sharply in response to the nonprocessed carbohydrate test meal.

Table 3.1 presents an example of such a test experience.

**Table 3.1: FEMALE PATIENT, AGE 55, DIAGNOSED MULTIPLE
SCLEROSIS** Symptoms on arrival at the center: fuzzy vision and eye
muscle imbalance. Legs numb, walking difficult, feet droopy. Patchy
numbness throughout body. Diet: generally high in carbohydrates and
wheat products.

RESULTS OF A 6½-HOUR NONPROCESSED CARBOHYDRATE TEST MEAL

Hours	0	1½	2½	3½	4½	5½	6½
Fasting Blood-sugar Level	97	161	91	86	81	85	85
Lymphocyte Count	19			44			34

NOTE: Blood sugar level is determined by the number of milligrams (weight) of sugar per 100 milliliters
(volume) of blood. A level of 80–110 is normal. A rapid rise to over 200 within the 1½-hour time period
is one determination of clinical diabetes. Lymphocyte count is established by counting 100 white blood
cells in a blood sample, then categorizing these cells by type. Hence a count of 19 means that 19% of the
white cells present in the sample are lymphocytes. Normally 20 to 40% of the white cell count consists of
lymphocytes. However there should not be a marked increase in lymphocytes from the fasting state unless
there is a stress problem.

The rapid rise of blood sugar level (from 97 to 161), followed
by a precipitous decline (from 161 to 81) is popularly known as a
hypoglycemic reaction (hypo = low, glyc = glucose (sugar),
emia = blood, i.e., low blood sugar). Glucose is the usual form
in which carbohydrate is assimilated, and the hypoglycemic reaction indicates this person's system for metabolizing sugars is not
functioning well.

There are three factors involved in the body's system for
regulating the metabolizing carbohydrates.

1. *Speed of absorption.* Simple carbohydrates such as table sugar and fruits are made up of simple molecules that can easily and rapidly be absorbed into the blood when eaten. Complex carbohydrates, such as potatoes, rice, and millet, are made up of chains of molecules that must be broken down within the intestine into the more simple individual units before they can be absorbed. Therefore, when one eats complex carbohydrates, this breaking down process takes time, hence the "sugar" arriving in the bloodstream is distributed over time, regulating the impact on the system. On the other hand, simple carbohydrates are absorbed more rapidly and therefore must be handled by your system all at once.

2. *Conversion and assignment.* The digested food absorbed from the intestines is taken up by the blood vessels surrounding the intestines which form the portal vein. The portal vein transports this digested food directly to the liver, where the blood is filtered and the nutrients sorted out. If the liver is functioning well, the body's immediate needs for "sugar energy" will be released into the blood for transport to the site of need, and the remainder will be stored for later use. When the liver's normal function has been distorted, the regulation has been disturbed and it dumps large quantities of unneeded glucose into the blood. Blood tests reveal this by rapidly elevating blood sugar levels immediately after ingestion of simple carbohydrates.

3. *Operational monitoring.* The level of glucose in the blood as a result of this liver activity is subsequently monitored by the pancreas. Endocrine cells within the pancreas called the Islets of Langerhans secrete insulin, a hormone that interacts with glucose and removes it from the bloodstream by the process of metabolism. If pancreatic secretion of insulin is abnormally slow, blood glucose levels will rise sharply in the early hours after sugar intake. Later, as the insulin secretion finally arrives on the scene, blood glucose levels begin to fall as the insulin acts.

The case study illustrated by Table 3.1 is a typical example of malfunction of the liver/pancreas system for regulating blood sugar level. The patient experienced nervousness, tremors, sweating, headaches, and varying degrees of unsettling feelings. The response often begins with a "high" from excess blood sugar producing nervousness and hyperactivity. As the blood sugar level falls, the person experiences fatigue and depression. During the fatigue stage, any weaknesses or stresses already existing in the body will be exaggerated by the general loss of tone and energy. Hence, patients generally feel an aggravation of their disease symptoms during this low period.

However, even more important to our metabolic rejectivity hypothesis is this patient's lymphocyte-count response. In this particular patient, her immune system reacted strongly to the influx of fructose from the natural carbohydrates. The lymphocyte count taken at the beginning of the test was 19 percent. After 3½ hours, following the initial rush of glucose into the blood at 1½ hours, the lymphocyte count has more than doubled to 44 percent. After 6½ hours, when the blood glucose level has returned to 85, the lymphocyte count is still at 34 percent. The body in general has two natural regulating systems to monitor glucose needed for action energy: the liver, for conversion and assignment according to need, and the pancreas/insulin response, for metabolism and body tissue utilization. When both of these do not function in a balanced and complementary way, it appears that the body begins to identify glucose as an "unwanted substance" and calls the immune system, with its lymphocytic scavenger forces, in to make a final stand. This response can occur with any food that the body considers, in its innate wisdom, as "unwanted foods."

During the one-at-a-time Response Diet food testing, another phase of the Kaslow program, this patient also discovered a nontolerated response to broccoli! Habitual eating of broccoli therefore was adding to the immune system response an additional signal beyond the nonprocessed carbohydrate meal of the existence of a glucose-regulation failure. As a result of regular intake of simple carbohydrates and broccoli, an intensified challenge to the immune-system responses was causing this patient constant internal distress, further fatiguing already distorted self-regulation systems. Exhaustion finally resulted from the system's long-term effort to cope with onslaughts of unwanted substances, and a symptom complex we call a "disease" brought this patient to a doctor to seek help.

In this case, elimination of broccoli from the diet, careful choices of carbohydrates, plus modest vitamin and mineral supplementation to augment the efficiency of the liver/pancreas turned the situation completely around. The unwanted substances no longer threaten the normal metabolic pattern of her body. This patient now walks normally, has good use of her arms, and enjoys greatly improved vision.

Figure 3.1 presents another example of this combination of the rejectivity immune-system reaction to the nonprocessed carbohydrate test.

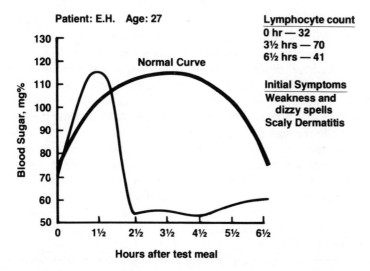

Figure 3.1:   BLOOD-SUGAR AND LYMPHOCYTE RESPONSE TO NONPROCESSED CARBOHYDRATE TOLERANCE TEST

The sequence of events shown in Figure 3.1 indicates that the patient's liver regulation of glucose was not functioning adequately to accommodate the large intake of fruit and very rapidly passed a surplus of glucose into the blood. The blood glucose level rose from a normal level of 70 to that of 115 within 1½ hours. During this period, the pancreas would under normal conditions have released adequate insulin to control the rising blood sugar levels, but this system also seemed to be functionally impaired. At 2½ hours, there is a strong attempt by the body to control this sudden elevation of blood glucose and the immune system is alerted to send out lymphocytes to begin the task of scavenging.

By 3½ hours, the lymphocyte count, which had begun at 32, jumped to 70, indicating a strong response by the immune system to an "unwanted" substance, and the blood glucose is reduced to about 53 mg. percent.

DISTORTION OF SELF-REGULATION

In the following chapter we explore the many systems within the body that are constantly active in the monitoring and maintaining of essential life activities. Activities we are more aware of are breathing, flushing, heartbeat rate, and perspiration. Activities we are little if at all aware of, such as digestion and metabolization of foods, cell building, and internal-damage repair, are directed and managed by innate self-regulation systems built into the body through the evolutionary process.

In the examples we have just been examining, we can see that the body has an elaborate self-regulation system for the intake, absorption, metabolization, monitoring, and utilization of glucose—the energy "fuel" for action. When function is normal, the human body *knows* how much glucose it needs, how to regulate its intake and use, and how to store surpluses for later use or excrete them.

There is a primary system, the liver, that makes decisions about how much glucose to release into the bloodstream for delivery to action centers, how much to store, and how much to secrete. The first back-up system is the pancreas, which keeps track of blood sugar levels and releases the appropriate amount of insulin to counterbalance any significant surplus of glucose that may be passed on by the liver. The second back-up system is apparently the immune system. If both the liver and the pancreas are unsuccessful in their efforts to manage the unwanted glucose or other substances in the body, the self-defense system rises to the occasion, identifying surplus glucose or other substances as unwanted. The lymphocytes are sent forth to initiate a signal-symptom system to alert the person and remove from the bloodstream those products unacceptable to the individual's well-being.

In the two patients we discussed earlier, Diane and Bonnie, and in hundreds of additional cases, it is apparent to us that this entire metabolic process has become confused. Patients' natural self-regulation systems for the metabolization of carbohydrates into glucose, at least by our test meal, and the subsequent management as well as utilization of glucose within the body have been seriously distorted. From the patients' personal experiences during the test periods, it is very apparent that this distortion and failure of the body's system for successful food metabolism is directly related to the diagnosed "disease" that brought them to the Center for treatment.

William H. Philpott, M.D., of the Ecology House Clinic in Oklahoma City, is working along lines similar to our metabolic rejectivity hypothesis. In Dr. Philpott's article, "Methods of Reversing the Stimuli-Evoked Pancreatic Insufficiencies of Chronic Degenerative Diseases," he describes a scenario for malfunction of the pancreas similar to ours for the relationship between carbohydrate metabolism and food allergy responses:

> The pancreas emerges as the initial and most important stress shock organ. An overstressed pancreas adapts to this stress by inhibition of its own function, thus producing a selective stimulus evoked [by eating nontolerated foods] pancreatic insufficiency. As far as foods and chemicals are concerned, this pancreatic insufficiency adaptation can be identified as a state of addiction.

Since the individual continues to eat foods, despite the fact that the body cannot, for the most part, utilize them, there is an *adaptation* that is attributable to the *addiction phenomenon*. In our view, it is this addiction, the craving of foods which the body cannot metabolize, leads to metabolic rejectivity.

This raises the question: What is causing the distortion of the normally self-regulating metabolic systems? Based on our clinical experience, giving consideration to the body's metabolic and immune systems, recognition to the effects of chronic stress, and finally studying repeatedly the Diet Surveys completed by hundreds of patients, we have evolved a working hypothesis.

Changes in American food consumption patterns, increasing levels of stress, decreasing patterns of physical activity, and, most important, a recognition of food allergies and food rejection combine to produce the *Metabolic Rejectivity Syndrome.*

STEPS IN UNDERSTANDING THE METABOLIC REJECTIVITY SYNDROME (MRS)

1. In Chapter 5, we discuss the McGovern Report, an analysis of American food consumption patterns prepared by the United States Senate Select Committee on Nutrition and Human Needs, headed by Senator George McGovern of South Dakota. This report details the marked increase in America of consumption of processed, refined, and sugared foods over the past 50 years. Sugar consumption has almost doubled during this period, from 10% to 18% of total calories. Processed and refined foods have become the basic staple of the average American diet. Sugared and refined foods *do not contain* the many *vitamin* and *mineral elements essential to self-regulation in the body.* In Chapter 5, we explore how vitamins and minerals seem directly related to body maintenance functions.

2. At the same time that these foods habits have been changing, individuals in our society have been experiencing increasing stress. Environmental pollution, rapid social change (especially in family structure), "hot" military wars and "cold" political wars, the appearance of nuclear issues, and the inflationary economic upheavals are but a few of the personal and social stresses becoming more intense in our times. In addition, one of the body's natural methods of dealing with stress, physical exercise, all but disappeared in general American lifestyle habits until quite recently.

3. These nutritional and at times significant imbalances and the lack of awareness about the effects of stress ultimately have led to a persisting breakdown and the development of a distortion of normal body processes. Gradually, over the last few decades, an increasing number of people have reached the symptomatic "threshold" of their body's capacity to adapt to food patterns involving nontolerated substances, stress levels, and unfavorable environmental stimuli.

Once they pass this threshold, the liver/pancreas (insulin) system for storage and metabolizing carbohydrates becomes overloaded and fatigued. Gradually, many foods become a problem as the entire food metabolizing process becomes stressed and functions inefficiently.

4. Among these persons who are overloading the body's metabolism system are many with either genetic or acquired sensitivities to specific foods. When these food-allergy responses are added to the already-failing metabolism system, further confusion and degeneration result.

For each of these people with food sensitivities, there are specific foods that the body identifies as nontolerated, even though the food may be thought of as nutritious and beneficial. At the moment, we have no code with which to predict what foods are likely to be rejected by any individual, and there is no correlation of specific foods to a related disease.

5. For the sake of convenience of preparation, a major factor in American food habits, people tend to narrow down food choices to a relatively few "favorite" items. They then purchase, prepare, and eat habitually these few foods, many times a week if not every day. If one or more of these habitually eaten foods repeatedly trigger the body's immune responses—either as a result of genetic intolerance or acquired rejection—the body accumulates a biological list of *nontolerated* foods. In a sense, the body says, "I've had enough of this food, I need other foods to balance out my system. I will no longer tolerate any of this substance!"

6. Individuals, not relating food habits to the onset of the body's signals of distress, continue to eat these "favorite" foods. This is especially true if there is a taste addiction or an emotional attachment to the foods. If physical activity becomes limited by dysfunction, food choices may even be narrowed further for the sake of convenience. The effort required to go out to purchase additional foods and to prepare a variety of foods seems too great.

7. The body's list of nontolerated foods has identified certain substances as "unwanted, excess, or foreign" material, the trigger for the immune system. Thus, each time the foods are eaten, lymphocytes—the white blood cells that scavenge foreign bodies or clean up damaged tissue—are sent forth to remove the substance.

8. Habitual eating of nontolerated foods produces an almost continuous immune response. The immune system, designed to be episodic and to deal with emergencies, is used almost all the time and becomes fatigued. The lymphocytes try ever harder to accomplish their task, and the system dispatches ever-increasing numbers of them as self-regulation degenerates. The lymphocytes flood the bloodstream, especially after meals containing foods the body has rejected over and over again.

9. Soon after eating a large amount of unwanted foods, there are far more lymphocytes in the bloodstream than are needed to scavenge the unwanted food substances. These surplus lymphocytes, whose biological job it is to scavenge unwanted material or distressed tissue, seek a target. If there are stressed tissues in the body, the lymphocytes will find them. For any number of reasons in a person's life, including nutritional imbalance, unresolved stress is manifested in organs and tissues. Once the surplus lymphocytes have found such a site, they will harass the target tissue faster than the body can restore it. As a consequence, we have the onset of the process of a degenerative disease in the target organ. This target organ could be the synovial membrane of a joint, the myelin sheath of the nerves or the lining membrane of a blood vessel, such as the coronary artery.

10. The stressed area, or target site for the lymphocytes, sends out distress signals of swelling, pain, dysfunction, and inability to self-correct. We call these signals symptoms of disease. As long as the individual's nutrition remains unbalanced, the nontolerated foods continue to be eaten, and other emotional and environmental stresses go unrecognized, this process builds on itself, creating greater pain and dysfunction in the affected area. More and more scavenging lymphocytes are called into play in an increasing spiral of chronic degeneration.

As a footnote to this hypothesis, we add an additional comment about the relationship between distortion of the carbohydrate-metabolism system in the liver/pancreas and the overreaction of the immune system to nontolerated foods. This is somewhat of a chicken-and-egg story. Without extensive research, there is no way to tell whether the food allergies are significant in the breakdown of the carbohydrate-metabolism process or whether the failure of the carbohydrate-metabolism process makes the body more sensitive to nontolerated foods. The progression may be different for each person.

However, we do know from clinical experience that the two phenomena—distortion of carbohydrate metabolism and rejectivity of foods—are *both* observable in almost every patient experiencing chronic and degenerative disorders who comes to our Centers for care.

THE SAME PROCESS, DIFFERENT SIGNALS

Based on our clinical experience with this hypothesis, we propose that most chronic and degenerative diseases *may be the same disorder, metabolic rejectivity,* given different names because of the site within the body harassed by the overstimulated lymphocyte activity.

The reasons why selected target sites are distressed in each individual is not clear. In Kenneth Pelletier's book, *Mind as Healer, Mind as Slayer,* he discusses at length the correlation between personality characteristics and certain diseases. It may very well be that individuals focus the unresolved stresses in their lives in (unconsciously) selected organ and/or tissue systems.

From our clinical experience, we are assured that the site at which the symptoms appear is the warning signal of a general *body regulation failure* but this signal is *not the disease itself!* By this we mean that in chronic and degenerative diseases there are no invading agents that are causing the pain, inflammation, and dysfunction at the site of the symptoms, as is the case in infectious diseases. As we pointed out in Chapter 2, allopathic medicine has spent a great deal of time, money, and energy looking for these causative agents for multiple sclerosis, arthritis, cardiovascular disorders, diabetes, and other chronic diseases. It may very well be that none will ever be identified.

The following examples will clarify the notion that the symptoms of degenerative diseases are indications of the failure of the body's self-regulation system, not the presence of infectious agents.

Diabetes

This disorder of the maturity-type is right at the heart of our discussion, because diabetes is the result of a direct distortion of the body's total capacity to regulate carbohydrate metabolism. The entire metabolic regulation of the liver/pancreas system for managing glucose levels in the blood is "out of order" in someone experiencing sugar diabetes. Chronic accumulation of high blood sugar levels ultimately causes diabetic shock and leads to coma.

As we said before, insulin secreted by the pancreas controls blood glucose levels. However, many persons experiencing diabetes with elevated blood glucose levels also have *adequate insulin* levels in their blood. Therefore, the problem usually seems to be in the metabolic interaction between glucose and insulin in the bloodstream, not in a deficiency of insulin.

A recent review of diabetes research in *Science News* indicated that only 20% of diabetics are insulin deficient. Why does insulin in the remaining 80% fail to interact with glucose? In the *New England Journal of Medicine*, Michele Muggeo and C. R. Kahn report they found *antibodies* (emphasis added; these are stimulated by lymphocytes) attached to receptor cells. These receptor cells enhance the interaction between the insulin and the glucose. These antibodies prevent the completion of that interaction. According to our metabolic rejectivity hypothesis, we have found lymphocytes appearing as a reaction to food rejection.

Traditional medicine's response to this information would be to institute immunosuppressant drugs to suppress the scavenging lymphocyte production. This may diminish the effects of the problem but does nothing to solve it.

We ask, instead, where did that lymphocyte come from? Through rebalancing of nutritional input and elimination of rejected foods, we can stop unnecessary lymphocyte production, allowing the body to self-correct rather than making it deal with even further stress and distortion through drugs.

Our hypothesis is that abnormal metabolism of carbohydrates caused by persistent long-term nutritional imbalance as well as deficiencies is the precursor of the disorder called maturity-onset diabetes. The entire liver/pancreas interaction system gradually becomes distorted by repeated overuse of sugar, other simple carbohydrates, and processed foods deficient in needed nutrient

elements. Eventually, the person experiences a rejectivity reaction
to intake of simple carbohydrates—as the case histories reported
earlier have shown.

In certain individuals, the phenomenon of food allergy and
rejectivity is an added burden. In addition to the collapse of the
metabolic system for regulation of glucose, the immune response
to nontolerated foods floods their bloodstream with surplus
lymphocytes seeking a target. For some reason, these lymphocytes (or antibodies, if we think about the Muggeo/Kahn article)
may effect the receptor cells that act as the communication
link between insulin and glucose, blocking their interaction. The
result is what we have labeled diabetes, the most rapidly increasing health problem in the United States!

Phil P., a 40-year-old patient, came to the Kaslow Center
after living with uncontrolled diabetes for 15 years. Because of
persistent high levels of sugar in his urine, he was taking, under
doctor's orders, large doses of orinase, tolinase, and DBI (all
insulin substitutes) daily. His fasting blood glucose level was
269 mg percent (normal is 80–110) or higher at times. He had
totally eliminated his intake of table sugar as a result of previous
medical advice, but his intake of bread, dairy products, and fruits
in significant quantities had been *prescribed* by doctors as a daily
diet.

During the Response Diet food-testing process at the Kaslow
Center, Phil discovered significant rejectivity responses to fruit,
bread, and dairy products and to some vegetables. He eliminated
these rejected foods from his diet, balanced, using a wide variety,
his general food intake with acceptable foods, and started taking
a modest vitamin and mineral supplementation.

His blood glucose level dropped to 169 within a week and
has continued to moderate. Through active monitoring of his diet
he is now drug free, has no excess sugar in his urine, and feels
alert and robust again.

Multiple Sclerosis

The symptoms of the disease called multiple sclerosis involve
impaired muscular coordination, double or diminishing vision,
loss of bladder control (incontinence), difficulty maintaining
balance, numbness, and a host of other disabling symptoms.

All of these effects are the result of a disturbance of communication in the nervous system caused by deterioration of the nerve insulation, or myelin sheath. Messages between the brain and internal actions systems become garbled and misinterpreted, interfering with routine body action.

For some reason, people experiencing multiple sclerosis focus their particular body stresses in the myelin sheath membrane surrounding the nerves, causing swelling in this coating. The metabolic-rejectivity-stimulated lymphocytes, seeking a target, harass these myelin membranes. When the process becomes chronic, the signals resulting from this activity suggest multiple sclerosis, and an examination of the myelin tissues confirms the diagnosis.

Linda Dunlap now of the Kaslow Center in Newport Beach, California, and Diane Mogul now of the Kaslow Center in San Diego, California, are but two of the hundreds of patients who have come to Santa Barbara diagnosed as afflicted with multiple sclerosis.

By response diet testing to find and remove rejected foods, rebalancing nutritional intake to provide needed elements, recognizing significant stressful situations, and improving body movement and oxygen utilization, Linda and Diane are part of the large majority of other multiple sclerosis patients who have come to the Kaslow Center in Santa Barbara, California, to return to a life free of dysfunction and distress. If someone is willing to maintain the program once begun and the body is free of the distorting factors affecting natural self-regulation, *the body knows how to heal itself!*

Rheumatoid and Osteoarthritis

Rheumatoid arthritis involves the synovial membranes that secrete a fluid lubricating the skeletal joints. Rheumatoid arthritis is an inflammation of the synovial membrane, reducing the liquids that act as lubricants. Osteoarthritis results from pathologic changes and malformations of the bony structure of the joints, and at times these malformations irritate the synovial membranes. The signals of arthritis are swelling, stiffness, and pain in skeletal joints and at times redness of the joints.

Again we say that these signals are indicators of distress in the natural self-regulation systems in the body. Under normal function states these systems provide the lubricating fluid or manage the construction of bone. Our medical center surveys show that individuals experiencing arthritis will tend to focus their long-term emotional stress or concentrate their physical stress in the muscles and joints.

The process we have described as the Metabolic Rejectivity Syndrome from foods will discharge a barrage of lymphocytes, which seek their target in these stressed joints, and over a period of time degenerative changes occur which are labeled arthritis. The following illustration is drawn from a microscopic photograph of synovial membrane tissue surgically removed from a rheumatoid joint. Hundreds of scavenging lymphocytes have gathered at the stressed site and degeneration has taken place in the joint structure.

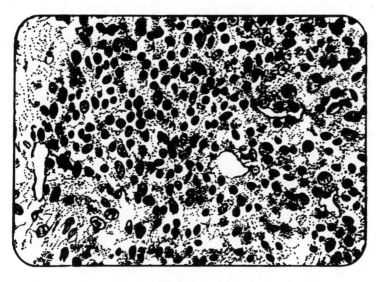

**Figure 3.2:   LYMPHOCYTIC INVASION
OF RHEUMATOID SYNOVITIS**

Bonnie S., age 40, was very overweight (obesity is commonly found in combination with arthritis) and severely disabled by rheumatoid arthritis. She didn't like having others "care for her" and resisted taking drugs. Bonnie failed to see that her daily six-pack of cola drinks might be related to her problems. Her weight had varied since her teens and was at 262 pounds when she arrived at the Kaslow Center in Santa Barbara. Her doctors had told her she had an incurable chronic, degenerative disease and that she should learn to live with it. They also indicated that her intuitive interest in nutrition, supported by books from health food stores, was a waste of time and money.

Bonnie said as soon as she walked into the Kaslow Center, she knew she had "found it." "It" was a significant attitude change from the previously expressed perspective that she should live with her problems. She discovered through food response testing a bad reaction to eggs, a milder one to cheeses and wheat. Asparagus made her nauseated and gave her a headache.

Bonnie eliminated these rejected foods from her diet, gave up the six-pack of colas a day, rebalanced her nutritional intake, and began to exercise daily. Within four months, she lost 77 pounds. Motivated by her new feelings of freedom and mobility, she continued on toward her goal of losing 140 pounds and being able to walk as much as 5 miles a day.

Bonnie is one of several hundred patients who have come to the Kaslow Centers seeking relief from arthritis. Those who have been willing to devote the time and effort to testing for nontolerated foods, designing a balanced diet, identifying and relaxing emotional stress, and embarking on a continuing exercise program have found freedom from pain and dysfunction.

Cardiovascular Disorders

There are two basic categories of cardiovascular disorders: hypertension and atherosclerosis.

Hypertension is a name for high blood pressure and does not necessarily mean that persons experiencing hypertension are always tense and nervous. Instead, it means that their blood pressure, which would normally measure at a high (systolic) of 120 to 140 and a low (diastolic) of 70, may remain at higher figures even when they are resting.

When we exercise or exert our body, the blood pressure rises to keep nutrients and oxygen flowing to the active muscles. After our blood pressure reaches its upper limits and we continue to exert, the body goes into "oxygen debt" and we begin to pant for breath and experience a pounding heart. A person with hypertension lives constantly in a state closer to those upper limits, creating a greater risk of crisis in the cardiovascular system.

Atherosclerosis results from the accumulation of damaged or scarred tissue (plaque) on the walls of the arteries throughout the body. Sites of this damage can block blood flow and diminish the proper circulation of nutrients and oxygen throughout the body.

If atherosclerosis blocks the arteries that supply blood to the heart muscle itself, the disorder is usually called coronary artery disease. A crisis caused by blockage of blood flow through these coronary arteries by atherosclerosis is popularly called a "heart attack" or "coronary."

If blood flow is interrupted through the arteries supplying the brain, either by atherosclerosis or clotting, this is referred to as a "stroke." Strokes are frequently the result of a combination of hypertension and atherosclerosis. When the blood pressure is abnormally high and a severe blockage occurs, the result can cause a "blow-out" of the arterial system leading to the brain. The interruption of blood flow to the brain causes an immediate lapse of consciousness.

If one is to believe the massive flow of data stimulated by the low-cholesterol-diet promoters, excess cholesterol is the villain in most heart disorders. On closer examination, we find that the overloading of the body's capacity to metabolize simple carbohydrates (sugar) is more directly involved. Dr. Linus Pauling, in a newsletter of the Linus Pauling Institute, agrees that sugar, not fat, is the culprit:

> Coronary disease, which because of its striking symptoms would surely not have been ignored by physicians of earlier centuries, seems to be a disease of modern times. It has been reported in the medical literature only during the last 100 years. The increasing incidence of the disease closely parallels the increasing consumption of sugar. It is not at all correlated with the consumption of animal fat (saturated fat) or of total fat.
>
> John Yudkin, M.D., Ph.D., Emeritus Professor of Nutrition at London University, quotes several studies that indicate strongly that sucrose (table sugar), not animal fat, is

the villain in heart disease. Dr. A. M. Cohen in Jerusalem found that Yemenite Jews who had been in Israel only ten years or less had very little coronary disease, whereas those who had been in Israel 25 years had a high incidence of the disease. In the Yemen, their diet had been high in animal fat, but low in sugar, and in Israel they adopted the high sugar diet of that country.

Our hypothesis that the gradual failure of the body's capacity to metabolize simple carbohydrates, aggravated by the immune system's response to rejected foods, will cause degeneration of sites targeted by the immune system's lymphocytes is supported by Pauling's observation and our clinical experience with cardio-vascular patients. In these cases, the harassed sites in the body are the walls of the arteries. Figure 3.3 shows the accumulation of lymphocytes in the coronary artery removed from a patient who underwent a surgical procedure called a "coronary by-pass."

Some heart disease patients who come to the Kaslow Centers have previously tried special low-cholesterol diets and special exercise programs. One such program is described in *Live Longer Now* by Jon N. Leonard, J. L. Hofer, and N. Pritikin. This book

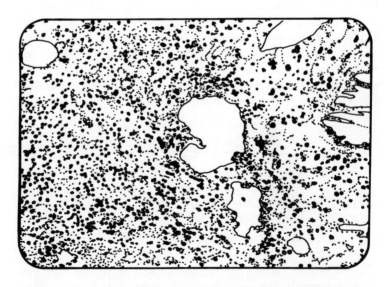

Figure 3.3: LYMPHOCYTIC INVASION OF CORONARY ARTERY

outlines a *prescribed diet* and exercise program containing many worthwhile suggestions, one of which is that "luckily for anyone who would like to stay healthy, a great deal can be done to prevent and reverse degenerative diseases with what we know right now. All that is needed is care in what one eats and how one exercises one's body. It is as simple as that."

From our point of view, the one major oversight in such a program is the lack of recognition of food rejectivity. *Limiting food choices by using prescribed diets increases the risk of rejectivity.* And, if the diet should include foods the person is already rejecting, the person's response to the diet could seriously worsen the situation.

Cardiovascular patients at the Kaslow Centers who have undertaken food rejectivity testing, balanced their nutritional intake (such an approach would include elimination of table sugar, reduction of simple carbohydrate intake, and moderation of fat intake), and begun an appropriate program of exercise and movement have experienced revitalization of the body and gained freedom from the restrictions of a "bad heart."

We have seen in the cases of diabetes, multiple sclerosis, arthritis, and cardiovascular disorders that a similar chain of events, the Metabolic Rejectivity Syndrome, is causing widely different signals (symptoms) depending on the stressed site chosen by the overstimulated lymphocyte response. Therefore, even though these disorders have been given different names according to the part of the body which is distressed, our hypothesis suggests that they are all essentially the same disorder—cumulative failure of the self-regulation systems of the body brought on by breakdown of the process for metabolizing carbohydrates through the liver/pancreas system, aggravated by overstimulated immune responses caused by habitual eating of foods that the body rejects.

Our clinical experience also indicates that many other disorders, ranging from clinical depression, hyperkinesis and schizophrenia (among the psychological illnesses) to psoriasis, colitis, and migraine among the physical illnesses, may result from Metabolic Rejectivity as well.

When patients undertake our program of food testing, nutrition balancing, and "getting moving again," many such disorders simply go away as the natural healing processes take over.

STAGES IN FOOD ALLERGY LEAD
TO METABOLIC REJECTIVITY

Dr. Hans Selye, whose pioneering work in the mid-1930s introduced what is now the widely recognized concept of the body's
response to repeated stress, outlines three stages in stress response:
initial response, general adaptation, and fatigue.

In terms of food allergy, the first stage—response—is the
most commonly recognized, e.g., hives, rashes, runny nose, or an
early symptom that appears when one eats a food one is "allergic
to." If someone is exposed to this food only occasionally, the
body will respond, the episode will pass, and the body will
regain its natural balance.

On the other hand, should such a substance be eaten regularly, the body tries to adapt to this stress. Recognizing that this
substance is a regular visitor, the body's internal regulation
system accommodates. As an analogy, if the weather became
consistently colder, you might set your thermostat higher. However, once you have set the thermostat higher, you become
accustomed to the new warmth, and you will feel chilly should
the temperature fall even slightly. This, in a way, is *addiction.*
You now need a slightly higher temperature in your environment
in order to feel normal.

The same thing happens with food allergies. Just as you may
crave alcohol and cigarettes, both of which produce immediate
body effects when used, your body can accommodate itself to
an allergic food and *learn to crave it.* Once the self-regulation
system is distorted by this continuing stress, it sends conflicting
signals to the brain. The foods you feel you need the most (sugar,
for instance) may be the culprits most responsible for the
problems.

Thus, the second stage of food allergy is adaptive *addiction*
to foods your body does not really want, a condition similar to
alcohol, drug, or cigarette addiction.

Eventually the body can stand it no longer and enters the
third stage: fatigue of the body response systems. This third
stage, in our view, is metabolic rejectivity. The immune system
becomes involved and the lymphocytes are sent forth. However,
because the entire system by now is in the fatigue stage, it is a

last ditch attempt by the body's immune response. The body then gives out intense signals to indicate that this food does not support the health of the body as nature intended.

In Dr. Marshall Mandell's book, *Dr. Mandell's 5-Day Allergy Relief System,* he refers to this process:

> Some allergies depend on the amount of exposure to a food, beverage, inhalant, or chemical. If you have an allergy to, say, corn and you eat corn in some form once a week, you may not have any reaction to it. But, if you eat corn flakes for breakfast, corn bread for lunch, and corn on the cob for dinner, with cornstarch in your dessert, you may build up a whopping reaction. This is why some patients say to me, "Bread bothers me, but not all the time. If I eat it for four or five days, I get into trouble. If I stop eating it, I am all right again, and can eat it again." What these patients are really saying is that they build up a specific level for four or five days and have cumulative symptoms; if they then discontinue eating bread, the overload of the wheat or yeast allergen drops down very quickly so that they can tolerate it again in this *cyclic* kind of pattern.
>
> On the other hand, you have a type of allergy in which you eat the same foods quite frequently and have developed an allergic type of addiction. Most people with food addictions are completely unaware that this process is taking place in their body. If a person misses a meal that would normally include the food to which he is allergic/addicted, withdrawal symptoms appear. In order not to experience the discomfort of a withdrawal reaction, the person actually has to keep eating the food to which he is allergic in order to stave off withdrawal symptoms.
>
> The third type of reaction is one in which you have a fixed reaction to a food. Every time you eat it, you react. It doesn't matter whether you have eaten the food along with another food, or whether you have only a small amount, you react. [Our hypothesis of MRS is that foods are now in this third stage manifesting metabolic rejectivity. The immune system has learned to identify them as nontolerable, and lymphocytes are actively scavenging these substances.]

One of the key signs that an allergy or allergy-like condition due to external factors may be present is the *reversibility* of the symptoms. After all, if a person has a rather severe nasal allergy to cat dander and gets a heavy exposure to a cat, the person's nose will probably itch or sneeze considerably. When either the person or the cat goes away, the aforementioned symptoms will begin to clear.

Bio-ecologic physicians know that one should not eat the same food over and over again for days at a time. Eating this will probably lead to a loss of tolerance for the frequently eaten food, which will then show up as an allergic or addictive reaction.

Thus we see that underneath all this overburdening of the body by food rejectivity, unbalanced nutrition, stress, and the feelings of hopelessness (discussed earlier), there exists a functional, healthy system with the power *to restore itself*, if we will but remove the overload.

Identifying rejected foods and removing them from the diet, assuring effective and balanced nutrition to meet the body's needs, alleviating stress, stimulating the body by appropriate exercise, and adopting an attitude that *you* are in charge of a healthy body all *support* the natural self-regulating and self-healing systems within your body. Once they are supported, *they know what to do* to heal any malfunction.

SOME COMPARATIVE VIEWS

It seems obvious then to ask, "If this process is so simple, how come more doctors and clinics are not aware of your approach?"

As we have discussed in Chapter 2, traditional medicine has remained within the purview that chronic disease is similar to infectious disease: Chronic disease is caused by invasion of the body by outside entities.

Our clinical experience has shown that almost all seriously chronic dysfunctions of the body can be traced primarily to the activity of abnormal carbohydrate metabolism or to some other food rejectivity, that is, the Metabolic Rejectivity Syndrome.

Because medical science has not looked at disease as an inter-related process but focuses instead on finding the invaders, there has been little, if any research done on this hypothesis. In addition, science seems to have almost forgotten the physiological concept of homeostasis, or natural self-regulation, and therefore has ignored the possible consequences of long-term distortion of this regulation (see Chapter 4).

At the Kaslow Centers we operate as observant clinicians, not laboratory technicians. Our interest is more in the improvement of the patient's life capabilities than in proving what is "right" or what is happening at the microscopic biochemical levels of the body. The Metabolic Rejectivity Syndrome may help to explain many disorders and diseases and we welcome any exploration of all possible explanations. With clinical patients, it seems only appropriate that these explorations center on the systemic and homeostatic levels of the body process, rather than at the isolated, structural/cellular levels of laboratory research.

Recently there have appeared in print a number of "nutritional" approaches to chronic and degenerative disease. Other than those of Drs. Mandell, Philpott, Randolph, and the other bioecologic and food allergy physicians, most of these approaches, for example, the Atkins diet, the Pritikin diet, the Swank diet, the low-cholesterol diets, have been prescriptive and designed to *treat the disease.*

These researchers have looked to the symptoms of each disease, or the patterns of the disease, and have designed specific diets to manipulate or modify those symptoms. For instance, since cholesterol was seen as the villain in heart disease, low-cholesterol or no-cholesterol diets were devised to alleviate or prevent heart disease. Since many multiple sclerosis patients have severe reactions to wheat and dairy products, diets have been devised excluding these substances, *without taking the Metabolic Rejectivity Syndrome* into account.

The difficulty with these prescriptive approaches, in our view, is that they assume all human bodies are the same, like automated chemical factories. They also do not recognize food rejection as a principal factor in the problem.

Fixed diets that are beneficial for some people may be disastrous for others. The Kaslow Program is an individualized plan providing each person with the opportunity to build for him or herself a balanced diet of all the nutrients the body needs, made up of foods that each person has experientially proven to be acceptable and nourishing to his or her body.

And, of course, food intolerance and rejectivity are at the heart of the Kaslow Program. In our view, any nutritional program for serious disease (and we include obesity as a rejectivity phenomenon) which does not take this factor into consideration has overlooked the most important key to distortion of the body's self-regulation and self-healing.

In addition to our ideas on metabolic rejectivity, the part of the Kaslow Program most essential to its success is the view that all education and treatment practices are designed to support the homeostatic self-healing and self-regulating systems of the body. Very few clinicians and researchers have given due regard to this basic attribute of the human organism.

As we did in the previous chapter, we will list some of the comparative assumptions of different schools of thought to clarify the bases of the Kaslow Program. (See next two pages.)

We applaud the many pioneers who are building public awareness of the importance of nutrition in disease and wellness. We would ask that they also consider an additional and critical factor of *metabolic rejectivity*—the nontolerance of specific foods, unique to each individual—especially in regard to those who are experiencing chronic disease.

Our clinical experience is that persons who come to understand the assumptions of the Kaslow Premise just outlined, who learn to identify those factors such as rejected foods which are distorting the self-regulating and self-healing systems within the body and change them, immediately begin to improve and continue to do so as long as they operate under these assumptions.

In the following chapter on the self-regulation process, we explore further how the body attempts to maintain health, how several stress factors—aggravated food allergies and nutritional imbalances, among others—accumulate to distort self-healing, and why the science of medicine seems to have overlooked this critical healing ability of the human body.

TRADITIONAL ALLOPATHIC MEDICINE	RECENT NUTRITIONAL PROGRAMS	THE KASLOW PREMISE
The function of nutrition is to provide energy for action and raw materials for body building.	The function of nutrition is to provide energy for action and raw materials for body building and to prevent disease by maintaining health.	The function of nutrition is to provide energy, raw materials, and *needed components of the self-regulating systems of the body.*
Disease may be caused by imbalances in nutrition, but this does not seem to be a major factor in the chronic diseases now being dealt with.	Disease can be caused by imbalances in nutrition, and this is the major cause of current problems.	Nutritional imbalance and *food rejectivity* are the principal distorters of natural self-healing systems.
The immune systems are somehow involved in most chronic disease. Drugs are given to suppress the immune response.	Immune system involvement is generally not discussed.	Metabolic rejectivity, the immune system's response to nontolerated foods, is a central issue. Nontolerated foods unique to each person must be identified and removed from the diet.
When disease occurs, the body is in error. Science must find the malfunction and fix it.	When chronic disease occurs, nutritional food choices have been in error. Science can prescribe a "corrective" diet to fix the body.	When disease occurs, natural self-regulation systems have been distorted by nutritional choices, attitudes, and stress. Identification of these distorters and the learning of new choices allow each individual

TRADITIONAL ALLOPATHIC MEDICINE	RECENT NUTRITIONAL PROGRAMS	THE KASLOW PREMISE
The proper approach to chronic disease is the use of drugs, surgery, and other external interventions to *attack* the symptoms of the disease.	The proper approach to chronic disease is to analyze the nutritional imbalances and develop a prescribed formula to *manipulate* the body and fix the disease.	to design a self-supporting program that allows the body to heal itself. The approach to chronic disease is to identify those factors that distort natural body regulation and remove them through patient education in self-management.
All bodies are essentially the same. Drug and surgery therapies should have more or less the same effect on everyone. Nutrition has a minimal effect and can more or less be ignored.	All bodies are the same. Nutritional formulas for each disease should work for everyone experiencing that disease. A person may remain on a fixed diet for an extended time.	Each body is unique. Each person must discover the special needs of the body and design a personal diet. Needs change; diets will change.
The patient is a passive receiver of treatment, a follower of instructions.	The patient is a passive receiver of treatment, a follower of instructions.	The patient is an active participant and learner, discovering those life factors that distort self-healing and learning how to change them and be well.

4

THE
AMAZING PROCESS
OF SELF-REGULATION

AS WE PROCEED THROUGH THE EVERYDAY ACTIVITIES of our lives, a staggering number of regulatory decisions are constantly being made by our bodies. Each of these decisions is guided by an exceptional "inner wisdom" built into the body by generations of evolutionary experience. This inner wisdom seeks balance, health, and preparedness for new action.

As discussed in the previous chapter on metabolic rejectivity, we have only recently begun to see the long-term effects of distortions of this built-in regulation system. If pressures accumulate to override or confuse natural self-regulation, chronic disease is an almost inevitable result.

Although we may not have thought much about it, each of us has direct knowledge of our own self-regulation processes. As an example, think about climbing several flights of stairs, reaching the top, and having to pause for a few minutes to get your breath and wait for your heartbeat to slow down.

When you climb stairs or do heavy work, your actions require energy, which is derived from the interaction of glucose and oxygen in the muscle systems. When the available oxygen in your body has been used or increasing demand is created for energy consumption, your breathing rate and heartbeat rate increase to supply more oxygen and glucose to the muscles. If you move too quickly or overexert, your body goes into "oxygen debt," your heart pounds, and you gasp for breath. The body signals you to stop using oxygen until more becomes available.

During this exertion, your body will begin to perspire. The exertion causes heat internally; in response the body turns on its cooling system. The evaporation of the perspiration from the skin cools you down. If you cool too rapidly or are exposed to a breeze, you may shiver: the body's attempt to regenerate some heat.

All of these automatic reactions are easily experienced examples of the built-in wisdom of the body seeking to restore the stability of all internal processes following any internal or external life event.

HOMEOSTASIS

In 1878, the eminent French physiologist Claude Bernard published his first paper on the "milieu interior," or environment within. Dr. Bernard was the first to explore the concept of homeostasis, which described the human organism as an *operating system*. Most other researchers of the time were concentrating on isolated cellular events. Bernard gave a great deal of attention to the human body's natural ability to self-correct and return to an internally balanced state whenever environmental or internal events forced a distortion of equilibrium.

Homeostasis, as defined by *Stedman's Medical Dictionary*, is "the state of equilibrium in the body with respect to various functions and to the chemical compositions of the fluids and tissues; e.g., temperature, heart rate, blood pressure, water content, blood sugar." This definition does not adequately emphasize the built-in regulation process within the body which consistently *seeks* homeostasis and in so doing responds to changes in body functions and chemical composition.

The strong inner drive toward homeostasis is manifest in all creatures, not just humans. Somehow, any animal's body knows what is needed to restore balance. Laboratory animals deprived of sodium for extended periods of time will naturally seek salt (sodium chloride). If several water dishes are placed in an animal's cage and only one contains salt, the animal will invariably approach the salted water and drink until its body's sodium level has been restored. The animal instinctively knows when the body needs sodium, where to find it among the choices presented, and, just as important, when that need has been met and sodium is no longer required.

The idea that each organism operates with this inner wisdom, although first presented in the late 1800s, has been relegated to the back shelf of medical knowledge. For example, all of the books listed below, found in a well-stocked public library, contain *no mention* of this basic principle:

> *A Complete Medical Guide*, Simon & Schuster, 1967
> *The Story of Medicine*, Golden Press, 1968
> *The Family Health Encyclopedia*, Lippincott, 1970
> *Schmidt Medical Discoveries, Who and When*, 1970
> *New Illustrated Medical and Health Encyclopedia*,
>   Stuttman, 1970
> *The Complete Illustrated Book of Better Health*,
>   J. G. Ferguson, 1973
> *Better Homes and Gardens Family Medical Guide*,
>   Meredith, 1973
> *Encyclopedia Britannica*, 1973
> *The Encyclopedia for Healthful Living*, Rodale Press,
>   1974
> *Collier's Encyclopedia*, 1975
> *The Rand-McNally Atlas of the Mind and Body*, 1976
> *Black's Medical Dictionary*, 1976

This is certainly not an exhaustive list of the currently popular reference works on general concepts of health and medicine, but it does indicate that the dominant germ theory of medicine affects what writers and editors consider important and/or unimportant.

A search of the Lane Medical Library at Stanford University, which includes the best in current thought in medicine, revealed one copy of one book, *Homeostasis*, by Maxwell Borow, M.D., published in 1977, which directly addressed the history and concept of homeostasis. The only other material specifically listed under this heading was a series of reports of symposia on homeostasis held in Europe during the 1960s. As far as we know, no such gatherings have been held in the United States.

We do not intend to condemn Stanford University or the publishers of the books listed above. We list this information to show the encompassing effect a narrow point of view can create on the limits of inquiry, research, and education. Where we look is certainly going to limit what we find. Science has been seeking adversarial invaders as causes of disease and has overlooked the issue of the natural healing power and wisdom within the body. Nature has been viewed as an adversary to be overcome, not as a source of self-regulation and healing.

We are indebted to Raymond D. Adams, M.D., a contributor to *Modern Home Medical Advisor*, for the following discussion of homeostasis and disease:

> The health and survival of the human organism as it moves around in its varied physical and social environment depends upon the maintenance of a stable fluid and chemical balance in all the vital organs of the body. *The precision of the physiological mechanics of the maintenance of this stability is almost incredible.*
>
> Temperature regulation, sleep, oxygenation of the blood, the levels of sodium, potassium, calcium, magnesium and all the essential chemical substances that maintain the activity of cell membranes are finely adjusted. The regulation of all these complex systems is through the vegetative nervous system, the central control of which is in the hypothalamus, a series of nerve cells in the center of the brain just above the pituitary gland, which controls the entire endocrine-hormonal system (thyroid, parathyroid, ovaries, testes, adrenal cortex, and medulla). At every level in this neuro-vegetative-hormonal system, *a change at one point results in compensation at another with constant feedback control.*
>
> Thus, one might conceive of man's nervous system as a great nerve and muscle apparatus through which information about the environment is transmitted through the sensory system to evoke movement of the organism and effect vege-

tative adjustment. Human instinctual and emotional reactions can always be viewed as having both an unconscious (visceral/internal) and a conscious (mental/external) aspect.

Persistent stimulation of the autonomic and vegetative systems *by stressful situations* may tax the organism's capacity to adjust and *give rise to functional disorders that stimulate disease* [emphasis added].

In Elmer and Alyce Green's book, *Beyond Biofeedback*, based on their work with psychosomatic illness at the Menninger Foundation in Topeka, Kansas, they point out another significant aspect of homeostasis as it relates to our interest in food allergy, addiction, and rejectivity:

> In a physiological sense, we could not survive without homeostasis, but it is important to know that continuous pressure can *modify homeostatic balance*. Homeostasis keeps us healthy and bouncing back from the strains and stresses of life—up to a point. If we are continuously reacting to stress, then homeostatic balances gradually shift, for they are not permanently fixed, and the undesirable result in our bodies is called psychosomatic disease. *If such a disease does develop, then homeostasis actively maintains it* until we do something about it [emphasis added].

C. Norman Shealy, M.D., a neurosurgeon at the Pain Control Clinic in LaCrosse, Wisconsin, describes this "adjustment capacity" of the homeostatic systems of the body as similar to a cup of water. We can take ⅓ cup of emotional stress, ⅓ cup of nutritional stress, and ⅓ cup fo environmental stress (or any combination of fractions adding up to one cup), but once the cup is full, any additional stress will overflow beyond the body's capacity to adjust, causing distortion of the homeostatic system throughout the body.

Thus, we see that persistent and continuous overstimulation of any process in the body can lead to distortion of the self-regulation system maintaining that process, and this distortion will then be reflected throughout the body, since all the regulation systems are irrevocably interrelated.

Once we have examined this view of the body, it is fairly easy to comprehend how persistent events such as food rejectivity, nutritional addictions or deficiencies, emotional stresses, and lack of exercise will each have their effect on the regulation of the body systems. As these stresses accumulate, and our adjustment cup runs over, chronic disease begins.

Since the term homeostasis implies a return to a fixed state, which never actually occurs in the human body, some theorists are now calling this complex interaction in the body "homeorhesis," meaning "the same flow," or "homeokinesis," meaning "the same action." These two words more clearly indicate the cybernetic flow of feedback and interregulation which actually takes place in the human body.

Whether one calls the process homeostasis, homeorhesis, or homeokinesis, our interest is in the intricate interrelationship among the many powers of self-control, self-direction, and self-management throughout the body.

HOMEOSTASIS, A CYBERNETIC SYSTEM

Within the last few decades, investigation of self-governing systems for computers and automated processes has given birth to the science of *cybernetics*. In a cybernetic system, aspects of the system are designed to identify operational difficulties or changes of course and to make automatic corrections to keep the system functional.

An example is the automatic pilot mechanism in an airplane. Once the course has been chosen and programmed into the system, the automatic pilot senses changes in the direction of the plane caused by winds and weight shifts such as fuel consumption or movement of passengers and continuously makes course corrections to keep the plane flying on course toward its destination.

The human body is a series of cybernetic systems, each feeding back management information to control points. These several systems are contained within a master system that manages the interaction among the several subsystems. It appears that the master system is in the hypothalamus, deep in the brain.

A map of these systems would look like a complex maze. On the wall of nutrition counselor Chelsea Reimer's office at the Kaslow Medical Self-Care Center in Santa Barbara is a chart about five feet wide and four feet high illustrating the biochemical metabolic pathways through the body. It is truly "amazing." It could be a combination of an electrical generating station's control board, a map of the New York subway system, and a diagram of a huge oil refinery all rolled into one. It indicates the many thousands of neurological and biochemical interactions and decisions taking place in your body as you read this paragraph. Figure 4.1 is a reproduction of just one small section of this chart, showing but a limited sample of the entire chart describing combination of sugars and fats with oxygen. And the entire chart illustrates only one of the many activities of the body, the metabolism of foods, not all body activities.

Let's take a look at some of these interwoven self-regulation systems to get a picture of this complex process.

The thinkers and planners. Our brain, central nervous system, and sensory organs are continuously processing information about our internal and external environment to make decisions about actions required for each life situation. Something as simple as putting the key into the lock on your car involves a series of interactions among your eyes, the touch sensations on the tips of your fingers, and your memory patterns about how the key system works, and the muscles of your trunk, arms, and fingers. All these interactions take place within seconds without any conscious awareness that they are needed.

The actors and movers. Involuntarily, the nerves and muscles keep the lungs breathing and keep the heart beating to circulate blood to bring in fresh resources and transport waste. Voluntarily, we use the nerves and muscles to perform every physical action of the body.

The catalysts and converters. Catalysts act as facilitators in the chemical breakdown processes in the manufacture of new chemicals. As we breathe air or ingest foods, enzymes, gastric acids, bile, vitamins, and a myriad of other body chemicals in

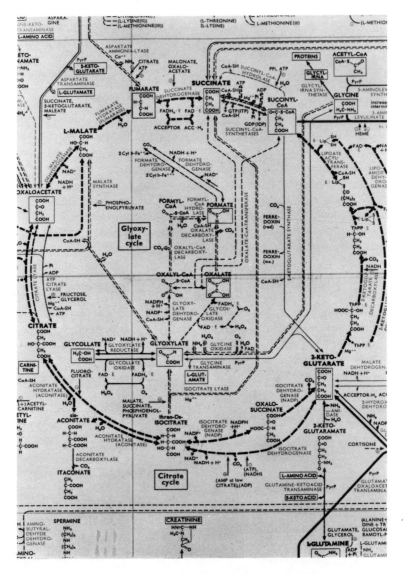

Figure 4.1:   THE GLYOXYLATE CYCLE

the stomach, intestines, and lungs break down incoming substances into basic elements needed for body functions. The liver/
pancreas system for carbohydrate metabolism, which we described
in Chapter 3, is an example. Catalysts and converters in the liver
and intestine change incoming foods into elemental body chemicals such as glucose and amino acids.

The carriers and messengers.   Individual body cells, blood
cells, the nervous system, and the glandular system constantly
carry information about bodily processes. For example, information about the temperature of the hands is relayed to the circulatory system notifying it to increase blood flow to the hands
when they become cold. Somehow this information flows from
cell to cell. It is not clear which cells simply transmit the information and which cells may participate in decisions about the
information as it flows through.

The builders and maintainers.   All cells in the body except
the brain and main stem of the nervous system are completely
replaced by the body within a seven-year period. In the bone
marrow and red blood cells, this process of supplying new cells
to replace worn tissue never ceases. The most obvious external
examples of this are the healing of skin wounds, continuous hair
growth, and the flaking away of old skin. However, all (with
the exceptions mentioned above) internal cells of the body are
involved in a similar renewal.

The filterers and excreters.   In the kidneys, liver, intestines,
and lymphatic system, incoming substances are monitored, selected
for inclusion or exclusion, utilized, stored, or excreted. The
simple act of drinking a glass of orange juice will trigger a series
of decisions about acid balance, glucose needs, liquid balance,
and possible need for the many chemical components of citrus
fruit. Based on current body status, these filterers and excreters
somehow know what to use, what to store, what to excrete. How
all this is accomplished is still a scientific mystery.

The scavengers and cleaners.   As tissue loses its vitality,
new cells replace old. White blood cells, the lymphocytic scavengers, come around to collect old or damaged cells and deliver

them to the excreters or remove them through the skin. As an example, a boil or pimple is an accumulation of white blood cells near the surface of the skin. When it bursts, the unwanted material is pushed out of the body.

The watchdogs and defenders. Toxic materials, infectious agents, or any other substances not wanted by the body are identified by "memory" lymphocytes (those developed from previous exposure, as is the case with smallpox vaccination) or basic DNA codes built into the genes. Once such materials are identified, white blood cells are sent forth to surround them and deliver them to the excreters. It should be mentioned here that this system is sensitive to *quantity* as well as to the quality of some substances. Trace metals, such as zinc, are essential to body function in minute quantities. However, larger quantities of the same material can lead to zinc poisoning, which may call the defenders into action.

The managers and regulators. Throughout this whole process, in ways we do not understand at all, the brain, the glandular system, the organs of the body, and even individual cells are constantly making decisions to try to maintain the vital healthy flow within the entire body process. All of the preceding examples are the result of some decisions made within the body in each of the subsystems. It is not known just how these systems interrelate and how these individual decisions are made.

All this activity is continuous in the human body, self-managed and self-regulated. The complexity and wisdom of this natural management system surpasses by many orders of magnitude the attempt science has made to develop computers, manufacture chemical substances, or create nuclear energy. Our attempts to intervene in this process to correct scientifically these self-governing decisions frequently cause further distress in the system. Our intervention can lead to a never-ending chain of side effects as we try to correct the problem we created through our previous action.

HOW DISTORTION OF SELF-REGULATION CAUSES CHRONIC DISEASE

Recently reported research examples indicate that some scientists are beginning to explore breakdown of self-regulation as a leading element in chronic problems.

When people become excessively overweight, we blame them for eating too much and think of this problem as a result of an emotional or hedonistic overload. Two University of Illinois researchers suspect something may have gone wrong with these individuals' chemical thermostats (most likely in the hypothalamus in the brain) that control appetite signals. Psychologists John D. Davis and David Wirtshafter believe the blood level of glycerol (a natural component of fat tissue) may turn on and off the body's desire for food by acting on special receptors in the brain. These cells signal hunger when glycerol levels fall and repletion when they rise. Although chronically obese people have high glycerol levels in the blood, their appetite signal receptors in the hypothalamus *may have stopped responding* to fluctuations in the substance level. In other words, when someone's glycerol monitor is not operating properly, the message indicating "I am full, I don't need any more food" is not received by the person, who continues to eat. The cliché "I just don't know when to stop" actually makes sense in this view.

This malfunction of a receptor cell sounds similar to the communication failure reported by Muggeo and Kahn in the insulin-glucose interaction in diabetics, discussed in the previous chapter. In that case, an antibody was found attached to the receptor cell, preventing communication. It would be interesting to discover whether antibodies are attached to the receptor cells in the hypothalamus of a chronically obese person.

In any case, people whose glycerol level receptor cells are not working will never get "enough" to eat. The satisfaction message from the brain which relieves their sensation of hunger is never received; hence they continue to eat beyond the needs of the body.

Criticism from others about eating habits may generate additional stress, which further distorts body messages and perpetuates the problem. Later in this chapter, we discuss the relationship between stress and self-regulation.

An additional example of self-regulation distortion in the development of chronic disease can be seen in the correlation between thyroid malfunction and arthritis. In almost every case of arthritis at the Kaslow Centers, we find a history of thyroid disorder. Dr. D. H. Copp of the University of British Columbia asks us to consider a connection between thyroid function and diseases that relate to calcium use in the body.

Investigation has indicated that the worry that a *healthy* person might take in too much calcium is perhaps unfounded. If an excess of calcium does accumulate in the body, overconsumption may not be entirely to blame. The person may be overstressed and we should look instead to a possible failure of the body's finely tuned machinery for self-control. Dr. Copp advises, "When calcium problems occur, rather than eliminating calcium from the diet, check first the body's system for dealing with calcium." One of the body's control centers for calcium is in the thyroid.

Too little calcium in the body can cause convulsions; too much can cause kidney stones, cardiac disorders, or contribute to arthritis. It is no wonder that the self-regulation system in the thyroid monitors the calcium supply so carefully that normal calcium fluctuations in the blood plasma are less than plus or minus 3%, regardless of intake or excretion.

It is sometimes difficult to relate a distorting factor directly to the regulation system involved. For instance, in the case of thyroid malfunction resulting in calcium imbalance or causing obesity, the distorting factor might range from iodine insufficiency (iodine is necessary for proper functioning of the thyroid), food rejectivity, or vitamin deficiency to continuing emotional overload. Only by achieving a general relaxation of all stressing factors can a reversal be achieved in a puzzling case. Science's perspective that each effect has a single, identifiable cause does not hold water in the interrelated and cybernetic world of internal regulation.

In both of these examples, we can see that an effect (obesity from overeating in the first case, accumulation of calcium in the second) is looked upon as the problem. Traditional medicine tends to manipulate these effects (weight loss through severe diet control in the first case, elimination of calcium from the diet in the second) rather than look behind them to the possible distortion of the body's natural self-regulation systems for managing the accumulation of fat or calcium. This distortion may be the true root of the problem.

Another tendency of traditional medicine, even if the cause were to be identified rather than the effect, is to want to fix the problem. As we have said before, the self-regulation systems are so interrelated and self-directed that attempts to fix them or direct their activity may very well cause further problems to arise. However, if we take the position that these self-regulation systems are essentially self-healing, then the task is to identify those factors that are distorting self-regulation and discover effective means to relieve these distortions. Instead of asking, "How can we fix the body?" we ask, "What is in the way of self-function?"

FACTORS THAT DISTORT
NATURAL SELF-REGULATION

Experience with hundreds of patients at the Kaslow Medical Self-Care Centers has shown us five central factors involved in the life patterns of persons with chronic and degenerative diseases which have resulted from distortion of their bodies' natural capacity to maintain health:

1. Habitual intake of metabolically rejected foods, resulting in aggravated food allergies (see Chapter 3).

2. Nutritional, vitamin, and mineral imbalances (see Chapter 5).

3. Stress and accumulated stress events (see the following section, this chapter).

4. Gradual loss of the body's vital capacity to utilize essential oxygen (see the latter part of this chapter).

5. Negative attitudes about the body, hope for the future (or loss of it), and personal power to determine outcome of life events (see Chapter 6).

Once the downward spiral of chronic disease begins, these factors become interdependent, intertwining to set up habits and life patterns which continue the degenerative process. At first, the person experiences disorder, or malfunction. Medical diagnosis may fail to pinpoint the problem or may sentence the person to a life of "living with" this "incurable" condition. The patient loses self-esteem, hope for the future, and any positive image of the body. The desire for physical activity is diminished as the person becomes ashamed of the body. Nutritional habits eventually concentrate on a few, easily prepared foods that are repeated regularly. When this cycle becomes well established, life vigor deteriorates and the individual retreats into inactivity, disability, and isolation.

Once this juncture is reached, any interaction with the world or new life activity is perceived as potentially stressful, and life itself becomes a major chore and/or a burden on others. If drugs or painful and expensive medical treatments are included, stress is increased exponentially. There appears to be no way out.

It seems difficult to believe that this degenerating body, capable of self-renewal, is just waiting for relief from the factors that are now a daily part of the person's routine.

In Chapter 6, on moving from helplessness to action, we explore the psychological and physiological ramifications of the loss of hope and self-esteem. The powerlessness experienced by those suffering from chronic and degenerative diseases is in itself a barrier to their renewal. As we describe the Kaslow Program throughout this book, you can discover how any individual can be empowered to act. At the Centers, each patient is surrounded by the attitude that he or she can and will get better through lifestyle changes and more productive personal choices based on the five factors that inhibit self-healing.

STRESS SHUTS DOWN THE THERMOSTATS

Professor Hans Selye of McGill University, Montreal, is the acknowledged father of physiological concepts concerning stress and tension. His first discussion of his now-famous general adaptation syndrome was published in 1936. In Dr. Selye's early work on stress, he thought in terms of the generalized physiological responses to environmental events.

For example, should you walk from a warm room into a cold room, the temperature change is a "stress" event on your body. Internal self-regulation systems will cause appropriate changes in respiration, blood flow, and heart rate, and will cause shivering and other body activities in order to maintain a constant internal temperature. Behavioral responses to the temperature change stressor might include putting on a sweater or turning on a heater. Both the internal self-regulation responses and the behavioral responses are strategies used by your body to respond to the stressor event.

Selye and others originally thought these responses were entirely physiological, could be experimentally predicted, and conclusions then drawn about how each stress event would affect the body. Recently, intervening factors have been explored that significantly affect human response: our attitudes, our fears, our emotions.

In Harold G. Wolfe's article, "The Nature of Stress in Man," he points out that in addition to actual physical interactions with the world,

> humans are further vulnerable because we react not only to the threat of danger, but to *threats and symbols of danger experienced in the past* which call forth reactions little different from those of an assault itself. We live lives so in contact with others and in such concern about their expectations of us that perhaps the greatest threat of all is our doubt about our ability to live the life of a human being . . . threatened by those very forces in society upon which we are most dependent for nourishment and life [emphasis added].

An external environmental event, or an internal, emotional memory event can turn on the body's stress response, activating the entire self-regulation system and changing a myriad of processes in the body. In general, if the stress event suggests immediate physical action, the internal self-regulation system will put food digestion, cell rebuilding, and other body maintenance processes "on hold." The energy thus conserved is therefore available for physical action. This is known as the fight/flight syndrome and represents our desire to flee a threatening situation if we can, or stand and defend ourselves if that seems necessary.

This reaction in the body is meant to be episodic. The self-regulation system is designed to meet unexpected threats from time to time, respond to them, then to relax and rebalance itself for readiness in future situations. The homeostatic principle in self-regulation returns the system to equilibrium. If, however, the stress persists as a result of emotional memory (worry) or an accumulation of environmental events, the response system remains turned on most of the time and is likely to become over-loaded and fatigued.

A good analogy for this process is that of a fire department that always receives a new alarm just as it is returning from a fire; there is no opportunity for the firefighters to rest, no chance to clean and maintain the equipment, and a growing sense of confusion and fatigue among the firefighters. Under these condi-tions, the entire system would soon collapse, equipment would fail at critical times, and firefighters would become upset and frustrated. Fire departments are designed to meet episodic emer-gencies and can fail if overloaded. The same is true of your body's stress-response systems.

Stress can affect the body's self-management in a number of ways, but there are two significant processes most likely to cause predictable distortion of the stress response system. We refer to these as "caught in a double bind" and "piling it on."

Caught in a Double Bind

Sara J., an attractive, potentially successful young woman of twenty-five arrived at the Kaslow Medical Self-Care Center complaining of chronic headaches, inability to sleep, exhaustion, and listlessness. A physical examination revealed no obvious disease that would cause this collection of symptoms.

She was living at home with her parents, worked intermit-tently at her father's fast-food chicken store, had few dates or contacts with peers, and followed a diet consisting mainly of chicken (of course), sweets, and snacks.

Sara was accompanied by her father. He had insisted on her visit to Dr. Kaslow and frequently spoke for her before she could respond to questions directed to her. Any astute observer could quickly tell that Sara was dominated by a caring, but doting father.

Sara's response to her father's attention was to try to keep him happy. However, this social behavior, which seemed appropriate when she began it as a child, was stifling her individuality as an adult. She had built up a strategy of avoiding her own need for personal integrity in order to accommodate to her father's dominating influence.

Her body was caught in the double bind of the unseen and unacknowledged stress and tension this strategy created. She wanted to react to her father's dominance (fight), or leave the home (flight), but neither action seemed permissible. Hence, her internal self-regulation system was in fairly constant alarm, especially when she was in the presence of her father. She lost energy and unconsciously chose sweets to regain it.

Response food testing revealed she was allergic to chicken, the main staple of her diet. The sugar, the chicken, and the continuing emotional stress placed ever-heavier loads on her self-regulation systems, which had given way to fatigue and begun to fail. She lapsed into headaches, insomnia, and listlessness.

It took about ten years for this process to build up in a strong, young body. This illustrates the elasticity and adaptability of the self-healing body as it attempts to maintain its balance and strength. Had she been older, in her fifties or sixties, this situation could easily have resulted in chronic, degenerative disease.

The attempt to restore homeostasis necessitated relaxation of the stressors and the design of new strategies for coping. A complete shift in her nutritional habits directed her to fresh fruits and vegetables, eliminated sugar, removed chicken for a while, and added some vitamin and mineral supplementation. Suggestions were made about peer activities, finding new outlets for her personal life, and establishing a new sense of personal identity. She sought work outside the family business. Perhaps to Sara's surprise, her father was ready for her to change and supported these suggestions.

In less than two weeks, her health began to improve. What had been a growing state of depression waned. She made new friends and found a job on her own. When Sara's system gained the nutritional elements it needed and was relieved of the metabolic rejectivity stress of the chicken, it took care of itself and she rapidly regained energy and vitality. Her headaches and insomnia disappeared. She regained her self-esteem and felt more confident about her abilities and future. *This new cycle was just as self-reinforcing as the depression had become.* Once started, it gained momentum.

It is important to mention here that there was no treatment for symptoms, no labeling as a "mental case," no mood drugs. Instead there was an identification of the factors that were distorting the natural self-regulation within the body and a program to allow the body to reestablish equilibrium.

There are many examples of people caught in the double bind of a job they hate or a relationship that is not productive. The conflict usually seems to rest between two choices, neither of which is seen to be permissible. A long-term failure to resolve such a situation places an overload on the stress-response systems in the body and fatigues the health-sustaining homeostatic process.

Piling It On

Thomas H. Holmes, M.D., of the University of Washington, has surveyed many thousands of people with serious illnesses. He discovered a high incidence in this population of recent (within one year) "significant life events." Some of these events were unfortunate, such as accidents or the death of loved ones, but others were "good," such as marriage, childbirth, or buying a new home.

Significant life events are all potential stressors. As shown in Table 4.1, Dr. Holmes assigned each type of event a point value based on the importance his interviewees gave them. An accumulation of a large number of points within a year or so was a good indicator of serious disease. In other words, the more significant life events a person experiences within a relatively short time, the more likely the person will become ill. People accumulating 300 points or more on this scale within the period of one year are considered to be in high risk position for illness.

Looking at the scale, one might fear that any significant event in life could lead to harmful results, thus causing one to

Table 4.1: HOLMES LIFE CHANGE INDEX

LIFE EVENT	SCALE OF IMPACT
Death of Spouse	100
Divorce	73
Marital Separation	65
Detention in Jail	63
Death of Close Family Member	63
Personal Injury or Illness	53
Marriage	50
Being Fired at Work	47
Marital Reconciliation	45
Retirement	45
Major Change in Family Member Behavior	44
Pregnancy	40
Sexual Difficulties	39
Business Adjustment	39
Financial Changes (up or down)	38
Death of a Close Friend	37
Change to Different Work	36
Change in Arguments with Spouse	35
Mortgage More than $10,000	31
Mortgage or Loan Foreclosure	30
Change in Work Responsibility	29
Son or Daughter Leaving Home	29
Trouble with In-Laws	29
Outstanding Personal Achievement	28
Spouse Beginning or Ceasing Work	26
Beginning or Ceasing Formal Schooling	26
Change in Living Conditions	25
Revision of Personal Habits	24
Troubles with Boss	23
Change in Working Hours or Conditions	20
Change in Residence	20
Change to New School	20
Change in Recreation Habits	19
Change in Church Activities	19
Change in Social Activities	18
Mortgage Less than $10,000	17
Change in Sleeping Habits	16
Change in Eating Habits	15
Vacation	13
Christmas (if approaching)	12
Minor Violations of the Law	11

Social Readjustment Rating Scale, by Holmes and Rahe, from the *Journal of Psychosomatic Research,* Vol. II (1967), pp. 213–218, reprinted with permission.

retreat from true participation in life. However, not all people who experience stress events in their lives become ill. The key is the strategy or coping mechanism each person chooses in order to deal with the stress events. There is stress in life. Without interaction and stress, nothing would happen—life would become dull and tedious. The question is "How do we recognize and deal with stress productively?"

If a person tends to *deny* (I'm strong, nothing ever bothers me), *repress* (I don't want to talk about it, it will go away), or *avoid* (I'll just let you have your way, it's not worth the trouble to work it out) stressful events, the stage may be set for later difficulties. The energy from these unresolved stress events will be held in the body, distorting the self-regulation systems.

In the Chapter 8 workbook we provide some simple exercises for recognizing and relaxing retained stress in the body.

COMING UP FOR AIR

It may be possible for someone to live for weeks without solid foods, for days without water or other liquids, but lack of oxygen will have significant effects within minutes. Oxygen is essential to all vital processes and is used by the body as it converts food into energy, builds and regenerates cells and tissue, and maintains homeostasis and balance. Anyone who has felt the rush of good feeling which can accompany a good, deep breath on a fresh spring morning knows the immediate and refreshing quality of oxygen. During any serious trauma, one of the first medical options is the provision of pure oxygen to revive body activity.

Some form of exercise is essential to proper oxygen conversion within the body. Not only through increased air intake but also through the stimulation of the entire lung/cardiovascular system, exercise increases oxygen potential in the body. Studies have shown that a person who exercises regularly can convert up to 50% more oxygen from the same amount of exercise as someone who is out of shape. That is, if a person who exercised regularly and one who did not ran 100 years side by side, the body of the person who engaged in exercise regularly would gain 50% more oxygen during the run than the nonexercising individual. This occurs because regular exercise expands the total capacity of the lung/cardiovascular system.

About ten years ago, Dr. Kenneth H. Cooper published his book, *Aerobics*, illustrating his work with groups in the Canadian and U.S. military forces. His concepts inaugurated the fads that have since become popular pastimes: jogging, bicycling, tennis, handball, and racketball.

The most effective aerobic exercises are those which involve all the major muscles of the body: the arms, legs, and trunk. These include running, swimming, brisk walking, and rope-skipping. Such exercise is continuous, rhythmic, and supportive of cardiovascular stimulation. Other exercises, such as weight-lifting, may build muscles but do not necessarily build cardiovascular endurance. Exercise such as tennis, golf, and bowling is discontinuous, involving only episodic exertion, which does not create a flowing lung/cardiovascular rhythm.

In *Aerobics*, Dr. Cooper explains the revitalizing effects of regular exercise on a wide variety of chronic disorders: heart disease, varicose veins, lung disease, smoking addiction, stomach ulcers, diabetes, obesity, back pain, arthritis, glaucoma, and psychological moods and attitudes.

Our hypothesis is that regular exercise and the increased intake of oxygen revitalizes the homeostatic self-regulation systems that have lain dormant and have been distorted by lack of adequate oxygen. This revitalization turns on the whole system and improves all body functions, changes attitudes, and stimulates new activities.

Anyone can exercise. In Chapter 8 we offer a number of ideas for building exercise into your daily routine, even if you are now limited by some dysfunction. Simply moving the body and breaking the old patterns of helplessness can revitalize internal processes. Deep breathing, even within a limited range of action, can bring badly needed oxygen into the system.

YOUR BODY KNOWS HOW

To summarize and review what we have been exploring in this chapter, nature has provided each human body with an incredible system of self-regulation which maintains health and vitality.

When chronic disease occurs, rather than seeking some outside agent to blame and remove we can look instead to those factors that can distort these systems of self-regulation. Working to identify and ameliorate these factors, we can prevent, reverse, or diminish this distortion, allowing the body to heal itself. Again, these factors are: metabolic rejectivity (aggravated food intolerance), nutritional, vitamin, and mineral imbalance, unresolved stress, lack of adequate oxygen, and limiting attitudes and beliefs.

The most important fact of all is that *all of these factors are under your control.* There is some action *you can take* to change the impact of each of these factors on your self-regulation systems and your life. This is why the Kaslow Program is called *Self-Care.* It is designed to assist you in the identification of the factors in your life which may lead to illness and to provide you with choices and ideas you can use to change these factors.

Nutrition is a key factor, one about which there are many conflicting views. In Chapter 5, "Good Food, Vitamins, and Minerals," we try to clear up some of the confusion that reigns about nutrition.

5

GOOD FOOD,
VITAMINS,
AND MINERALS

ONE OF THE VERY UNUSUAL STORIES TO EMERGE FROM
the Vietnam war is of interest to us here. The *Los Angeles Times*
reported:

> A study in progress under the auspices of the Navy's Center
> for Prisoner of War Studies suggests that the low-cholesterol,
> low-fat diet [rice and vegetables, also low sugar] of impris-
> oned Navy pilots contributed to their long-term physical
> health.
>
> John A. Plag, who directed the study, said he compared
> 78 former POWs with non-POW pilots who had flown
> missions over Vietnam during the same period as the POWs.
> Each of the pilots in the non-POW group was matched with
> a returned prisoner of war according to such variables as
> rank, marital status, years of schooling and number of flight
> hours. The control group agreed to undergo annual medical
> examinations of the same scope and complexity as those
> given the former POWs.
>
> Contrary to expectations, the non-POWs were less
> healthy. Of particular importance was a higher incidence
> in the control group [non-POWs] of cardio-vascular disease.
> When shot down, many of the POWs were well above their

ideal weight. On the reduced rations of captivity, which were undoubtedly lower in cholesterol and fat [and sugar, we might add] than the average American diet, many of the POWs fell to their ideal weight and remained at that level.

We note that even though the POWs may have dealt with some level of stress in the context of captivity, their daily life was essentially one of balanced nutrition, regular exercise, and minimum stress, compared to the daily regime of the non-POW pilots who were flying combat missions.

The main point of the article, however, is that the POW food was apparently "good food." Had someone told these POWs during their captivity that the diet of rice and vegetables was preferable to the American diet of meat, potatoes, thoroughly cooked vegetables, and dessert they had received on the carriers, they probably would have rejected the notion completely.

We have come to believe in the United States that meat, dairy products, grains and starches, and vegetables, with a good dessert thrown in to sweeten the tooth, are the components of "good food." Not long ago, the American housewife was assured she was preparing the best possible meal for her family if she placed a good portion of red meat, fish or chicken, a portion of mashed potatoes, and a vegetable on each plate, accompanied by a full glass of milk. This array has been thought of as "good food" and no doubt derives from the hearty farm meals looked on as essential from our not-too-distant history as workers of the land.

Even if most Americans maintained such a diet, there would be some problems, as noted in the Vietnam story. However, even *this* notion of "good food" has faded away as American eating habits have shifted significantly in the years since World War II.

EATING THE AMERICAN WAY

In the previous chapter, we pointed out how the medical concept of homeostasis has been overlooked in current medical thinking as a result of the prevailing notion of the single cause, or germ, theory of disease. Whereas homeostasis has been nearly forgotten, nutrition as a factor in health and disease has been repressed in the medical world. Only recently, in the public forum of books and magazine articles, has this issue come to the fore as a major factor in health. Paavo Airola, in *Are You Confused?* points out:

> There is virtually no independent nutrition research in the United States. Almost all research is done or sponsored by the commercial food industries involved in food production. The giant, billion-dollar food processing, chemical, and drug industries finance most of the nutrition research in the United States, both in private research centers and in the form of grants to the various universities. "He who pays the piper calls the tune." It would be naive to expect that the research paid for by these producers of processed, devitalized supermarket foods would reveal and condemn the real threat to the health of Americans: these same processed, devitalized and foodless foods!

In January 1977, The United States Senate Select Committee on Nutrition and Human Needs (now a subcommittee of the Senate Agriculture Committee) published a study, *Diet Related to Killer Diseases,* on American diets and how they have changed during this century. The report noted that six of the ten leading causes of death in the United States are linked to diet: heart disease, stroke, arteriosclerosis, cancer, cirrhosis of the liver, and diabetes. At the present time, these causes account for one-half of all deaths in the United States.

"American" food includes heavy proteins (beef and eggs), fats, refined sugar, refined and enriched flour, grains and cereals, mainly consumed in processed convenience foods. The growing dependence on these foods has emerged since World War II as the huge food producers, packagers, and supermarket chains have come to dominate food distribution in the United States. As this trend has grown, Americans have come to think of food less as *food* and more as *products.* Food processors also think of foods as products, and a number of key factors influence their decisions in food production and packaging.

Long shelf life. Foods that deteriorate during the time between harvest and customer purchase must be discarded and will bring no revenue. Hence, food producers seek to process, preserve, or otherwise package foods so that they will not be lost. Although waste prevention and efficient utilization are worthwhile ideals, the original motivation has been lost in a host of packaging and chemical additive schemes that remove food value and add substances the body cannot use.

Deterioration of foods in nature is essentially the result of natural combination of the elements in food with oxygen in the air. Hence, to preserve foods, processors may remove through refinement those elements most likely to combine with oxygen and add chemicals to inhibit oxygenation. Since digestion of foods depends almost entirely on the foods' interaction with oxygen, preserving the foods in this way has a direct and diminishing effect on food value.

Bright, colorful, and consistent physical appearance.   Consumers are conditioned by advertising and social custom to buy the brightest, cleanest, most uniform foods. Hence, food producers add colorings, stimulate uniform growth with chemicals and hormones, and cross-breed plants and animals for the sake of appearance alone. The producer can get more "square" tomatoes into a carton, and chickens with fuller breast portions sell better in the markets. None of this expensive activity increases the nutritional value of the foods, and the colorings and hormones are potentially toxic.

Convenience of preparation and consumption.   If there is one predominant factor in current American food habits, it is "fast foods." In the home we find slick, precooked and packaged foods ready to pop into the microwave oven. If one is too rushed to prepare food at home, there are an ever-growing number of "take-out" food stores offering chicken, hamburgers, french fries, and tacos. Almost all this food is deep-fat fried. Even in sit-down restaurants, most portions are prepackaged and processed, ready to be quick heated or grilled. A recent report indicates that as much as 33% of all foods consumed in the United States are purchased in restaurants or take-out stores. Unfortunately, fresh fruits and vegetables are rarely served in American restaurants and are not available at any of the fast-food outlets.

Promotability for impulse buying. American food producers have manufactured foods which did not even exist until recently: sugared cereals, corn and potato chips, prepared dips, processed cheeses, whipped oleomargarine, soft drinks, sugar-free soft drinks (a nonfood), decaffeinated coffee, enriched breads, dried and packaged soups, processed luncheon spreads, and on and on. Most of these kinds of foods are advertised heavily on television and displayed expensively in stores.

They are not foods. They are consumable products designed for high-profit sales in high volume, similar to razor blades, toothpaste, and cigarettes. The fact that the consumer eats them, hence, that they should have true nutritional value, is far down on the list of pertinent factors discussed in the planning and marketing of these items.

None of the four factors mentioned above, which dominate the thinking and planning of American food producers, leads to the distribution of foods containing the essential nutritional needs of consumers. We have marched away from fresh, natural foods and toward preserved, manufactured foods more easily controlled by the processor.

In addition, the refining and processing of foods as they are packaged usually involves "leaving out" a number of the vitamins and minerals so essential to nutritional value. This process starts all the way back at the farm when chemical fertilizers not containing the native mineral elements of the soil are used in place of organic fertilizers. The foods grown under these conditions contain less of the minerals and trace elements we discuss later in this chapter; for example, calcium, magnesium, potassium, and phosphorus. They also may contain less of the natural vitamin content.

Later, when the foods are "refined," especially the grains, more of these elements are removed, usually to make the flour more "white" and pure looking. Then, in hopes of making the product appear in a better light, the processor "enriches" the flour by adding some artificially manufactured vitamins. However, not all the original elements are replaced; thus the term "enriched" is somewhat misleading.

One item that is added to almost all processed foods is sugar. Processors know that Americans have a sweet tooth. Table 5.1

illustrates the content, by weight, of sugar in a number of processed foods. As we discussed in our chapter on metabolic rejectivity, this overload of sugar in the diet seriously distorts the liver/pancreas system for metabolizing carbohydrates.

**Table 5.1:   SUGAR CONTENT IN PROCESSED FOODS
(PERCENTAGE OF TOTAL WEIGHT)**

PRODUCT	%	PRODUCT	%
Jello	82.6	Cool Whip	21.0
Coffee-Mate	65.4	Libby's Peach Halves	17.9
Cremora	56.9	Shake'n Bake	17.4
Hershey Bar	51.4	Wyler's Beef Bouillon	14.8
Shake'n Bake (BBQ)	50.9	Shake'n Bake Italian	14.7
Sara Lee Choc. Cake	35.9	Dannon Blueberry Yogurt	13.7
Wish-Bone Russian Drsg.	30.2	Ritz Crackers	11.8
Heinz Tomato Ketchup	28.9	Del Monte Canned Corn	10.7
Quaker 100% Natural Cereal	23.9	Skippy Creamy Peanut Butter	9.2
Hamburger Helper	23.0	Coca-Cola (can)	8.8
Wish-Bone French Drsg.	23.0	Wish-Bone Italian Drsg.	7.3
Sealtest Choc. Ice Cream	21.4	Ragu Spaghetti Sauce	6.2

From *Consumer Reports*, March 1978 (256 Washington Street, Mt. Vernon, New York 10550), reprinted with permission.

When you are buying foods, read their labels. The ingredients in the foods must be listed in the order of their respective proportion in the food. If sugar is listed first, second, or even third, you can bet that the package contains a good portion of sugar, even though you might not think of the food as a source of sugar in your diet. Also, beware of dextrose, corn starch, corn syrup, and so-called "natural sweeteners." All of these are merely different names for sugar.

DIET CHANGES CAUSE SHIFTS
IN DISEASE PATTERNS

From a nutritional point of view, the most significant changes in the American diet in the past 65 years have included:

1. An increase in fat consumption from 32% of total calories in 1910 to 42% in 1976—related to rising incidence of heart disease.

2. An increase in consumption of simple carbohydrates (sugars and certain fruits) from 12% of total calories in 1910 to more than 18% in 1976.

3. A *decrease* in consumption of complex carbohydrates (starches such as potatoes, rice, some vegetables) from 37% of total calories in 1910 to 21% in 1976. Both the increase in consumption of simple carbohydrates and the decrease of complex carbohydrates are related to increasing incidence of diabetes and heart disease.

4. Beginning in the 1920s and 1930s the phenomenal rise in numbers of people smoking cigarettes established tobacco as a major product of American agriculture. This activity has been related to the escalating incidence of cancer.

These facts are summarized in *Diet Related to Killer Disease, Nutrition and Mental Health,* a book published by the Select Committee on Nutrition and Human Needs of the U.S. Senate, chaired by George McGovern of South Dakota, which has become known as the "McGovern Report" in nutrition circles. Information from this book has been analyzed and commented on in a booklet, "The Changing American Diet," published by the Center for Science in the Public Interest in Washington, D.C.

These data, indicating the overall shifts in the basic content of foods eaten in America, verify the results of the growing dominance of large corporate food producers and distributors. Not long ago, we thought "good food" was a good square "farm" meal. A meal of meat and eggs, potatoes or rice, a vegetable and dessert, with a glass of milk may be somewhat high in protein and fats, especially if it consists of large portions and is eaten by an individual living a sedentary lifestyle. However, these meals are preferable to the food styles now being adopted by the average American consisting of fried foods, refined and processed foods, foods with high sugar content, and diet lacking in fresh vegetables, complex carbohydrates, and essential vitamin and mineral elements.

WHAT CAN WE DO?

Should we go back to basic square meals? How can we figure out what makes up a good balanced diet in the midst of the mass of material now being published about nutrition? Do we need vitamins and minerals? Should we take food supplements? Are weight loss and other prescribed diets effective? These are among the questions many are asking as they try to sort out a reasonable plan for effective nutrition. Several approaches to answers to these questions have emerged.

The Formula Approach

Because Americans like to think in reductionist terms, we break everything down into its smallest possible components and analyze each detail. This approach to nutrition has been growing.

Looking at the body as a complex chemical machine, nutritionists who take the formula approach try to check out the myriad of activities in the body and determine the nutritional needs of each. From this, a very complex list of "needs" can be developed, similar to an inventory sheet to be checked each week or so to see what should be reordered.

Someone looking at nutrition from the formula approach can become obsessed with all these details, constantly checking to be sure that the body is receiving each of the necessary ingredients in just the right proportion. The health food stores thrive on these people. Every month or so some new "ingredient" is introduced which is supposedly magic in its nutrient power. Everyone should have it. Yeast, acidophilus, wheat germ, enzymes, etc., are all seen as necessities for the healthy person. Each vitamin and mineral is measured and monitored. A great deal of time and energy is spent organizing all the mental record-keeping on whether or not one is getting all the numerous individual items one needs.

One of the myths frequently shared by people who become interested in the formula approach implies that vitamins and minerals are, in themselves, foods. That is, if I have my protein drinks, stay away from sugar, snack on raw vegetables, and take my vitamin and mineral tablets, then I am eating a healthy diet.

As we discuss later, vitamins are coenzymes and catalysts (chemical interaction facilitators) in the process of food digestion and body self-regulation. They appear to function in the body most effectively only when in the presence of foods, acting in the digestion and assimilation process to promote the optimum use of the foods. Therefore, to take vitamins thinking they will supply food value is essentially a waste. Or, to take vitamins at times other than with foods usually means they will simply pass through the body without being utilized.

Minerals are among the basic elements of the earth and are taken from the ground by the plants we eat, and because some plants are used as animal foods, minerals are also an essential part of animal tissue. They are useful as food supplements only when the basic minerals needed by the body are missing from foods in the region or when specific deficiencies are discovered in the make-up of an individual at a given time. This introduces another approach to nutrition design.

The Deficiency Approach

Imagine a row of shelves on which there are hundreds of small jars, each jar containing one of the basic elements of life needed by the human body. Then imagine checking each of the jars every morning, or several times a week, to decide which elements you need at the moment to refill partially empty or empty jars.

Approaching nutrition from this point of view is a variation on the formula approach and is based on the identification and replenishment of deficiency. We have all heard conversations such as "I'm having headaches during my period, I must be low in iron." Or, "My constipation problem is acting up again. I'm not getting enough fiber."

Although these statements may have some validity, the assumption in this type of thinking is that each activity of the body is a predictable biochemical action. If we put the "right" material in, we can manage the process by formula and we can correct all of our problems.

Although a formula approach to nutrition may be preferable to drugs and chemicals in the possible solution of health problems, it has some of the same problems as a drug/chemical attitude. First, *you need an expert.* To use the formula approach, one must first have detailed knowledge of the present condition of your body and the abundance or absence of each element. Only then can the formula be prepared to meet your needs or correct your deficiencies. Every health food store, any number of nutrition teachers, evangelists of exotic and unusual diets, and even many physicians have their own schemes for assessing these needs and designing your formula. The assumption is that you know very little about your own body and that they can work out the formula just right for you. However, many apply their formula to everyone they see and not on an individual basis.

Second, *you become dependent on an outside assessment.* On some regular schedule you will have to reevaluate the levels of basic elements you feel you might need. The body is constantly changing. If you begin to take some supplement, say zinc, to replenish a supposed deficiency, you will not want to take zinc forever. You hope the deficiency will be replenished shortly and you will stop taking this supplement. But when? How do you know? You must go back and get more information from your expert.

Third, too frequently the people who assess your needs for these elements are also the people who sell them to you. This almost always creates a pressure to discover needs that may not be significant enough to warrant action but for which remedies are "prescribed" anyway.

This formula approach becomes very complex, dependent on outside authority, and expensive.

Still More Approaches

In addition to the formula approaches we have been discussing, the nutrition field has seen an onslaught of vegetarian belief systems, liquid protein schemes, weight-loss programs, and a host of books about magic diets and health foods, natural foods and organic foods.

Many of these ideas may have great value for individuals who seek them out to meet special needs. Problems arise when consumers try to gain some overall understanding of the issues so that they can make reasonable, effective decisions on their own. There is so much conflicting information, so many different approaches, and no agreement, especially in the medical community, about the basic issues. Statements from doctors and advocates of nutrition schemes range from claims for miracle cures to angry denials that nutrition has nothing at all to do with healing chronic disease.

Based on our clinical experience at the Kaslow Centers and the self-designed diets of successful Kaslow patients, we do know that there are some very simple concepts anyone can follow to overcome dysfunctions and illness and to promote general well-being and good health.

THE KASLOW APPROACH:
BALANCE, VARIETY, AND SELF-KNOWLEDGE

Recall our earlier story about the laboratory animals who were intentionally deprived of sodium. Instinctively, they sought out salted water to rebuild their deficient supply of the sodium. They had no professional authority to tell them they were lacking the necessary amount of sodium, no one to prescribe salt tablets. At some deep level within themselves, the animals know what to do.

This same level of knowledge and self-management exists in each human being. You can learn to be more in touch with your body's needs for certain elements and foods and also to identify those elements and foods that your body does not want and will reject.

Since the Kaslow Program is based on nutritional concepts, many patients and members of our lecture audiences ask, "What is the Kaslow Diet?" In our view, the assumptions on which this question is based represent a real barrier to the understanding of nutrition and health. This question implies that

1. Nutritional approaches to the prevention or amelioration of disease must be formulated to "treat the disease."

2. There is some magic formula science can develop to manipulate the patient's body back to health.

3. The chemistry of each body is the same. A formula diet listing prescribed foods for any given problem should be effective for anyone experiencing that problem.

4. Professionals are the designers of the magic formula, and the individual utilizing the diet should simply follow instructions.

5. Once the magic formula to correct a problem has been found, the person experiencing that problem may be restricted to that formula for a long period of time.

Interviews with patients and others interested in nutritional approaches to health have revealed that these views are held by many. The Kaslow Program is not based on any of these assumptions but on a completely different set of principles. In comparison to the five points above, the Kaslow Program assumes that

1. Nutritional approaches to chronic diseases should be self-designed to reduce or remove distortion of the natural self-regulation systems of the body. This is accomplished through identification and removal of rejected foods and establishment of wide variety in the diet.

2. There are no formulas for the effective treatment of each disease. The diet should address the condition and situation of the individual involved and be self-designed by the *person*, not the disease. Rather than attempting to overcome the disease, the diet is designed to rebalance and support the natural self-healing processes within the body.

3. Each human body is unique biologically. Diets designed for general populations will not work for many individual cases. Programs must be engineered to discover those particular aspects of an individual's life and nutrition habits which either assist or block the body's natural self-regulation systems.

4. The professional is a knowledgeable resource assisting the individual in learning how the body works and what nutritional plan will best serve that individual's needs.

5. Diets and nutritional plans should never remain fixed over

extended periods of time, especially if they are limited to a small number of food choices. Risk of food rejectivity is drastically increased if food selections are limited over a long period. With the Kaslow Program, people learn greater sensitivity to their own body needs and body responses and change their diets accordingly based on their intuitive knowledge.

The Kaslow nutritional approach is based on a three-step program aimed at teaching each person self-wellness and supporting the natural self-regulation systems of the body.

Step 1.   Removing Barriers to Self-Regulation

As discussed at length in Chapter 4, there are five major life-habit contributors to distortion of natural self-regulation; a nontolerance of certain foods resulting in metabolic rejectivity, a general nutritional imbalance, hidden or accumulated emotional stress, lack of an adequate supply of oxygen, and attitudes of helplessness and powerlessness are all factors that will distort the body's capacity to use foods effectively, even if one maintains a nutritious, balanced diet. Therefore, despite the fact that some of these factors might not be thought of as part of a nutrition program, we see removing any such barriers as integral to the success of a nutrition program.

Step 2.   Meeting the Body's Needs

There are basic elements—proteins, carbohydrates, vitamins, minerals, and trace metals—that each human organism needs to function in good health. These are available in a variety of foods. Without complex formulas, but with forethought and planning, all persons can design an appropriate and nourishing diet if they are willing to take the time to learn about themselves and their body.

In Chapter 8, you can learn how to put together light meals made up of a number of foods that will supply all your body needs. Heavy, meat-based meals made up of the "basic four" usually offer too much food and are also more expensive than these light meals.

A variety of vegetables, the light meats—fish and chicken— grains, nuts, and seeds, and eggs can provide a complete range of the basic elements needed by the body. The key is variety to assure intake of all the many elements and moderation to avoid overload.

Some vitamin and mineral supplementation may be advisable to counteract stress or during periods of recovery from serious illness, either chronic or infectious. We note again, vitamin and mineral supplements are not substitutes for foods. They interact with the foods you eat to facilitate the food's effective use in the body. If the foods you eat are unbalanced, or if you use vitamins and minerals as a substitute for certain foods, your system will not benefit.

Step 3. Individuality, Self-Knowledge, and Self-Management

The entire Kaslow Program is a series of surveys, interviews, and experiences designed to increase each person's awareness of those aspects of nutrition, life habits (time management, sleep patterns, worries and stresses), and attitudes which aggravate or diminish episodes of illness and/or promote feelings of well- being. There are no blanket formulas. Each person must seek understanding of his or her body and its unique experience of illness or wellness. Health and illness are personal experiences, not clinical entities with medical names.

Some people, because of a long history of conditioning and old attitudes, have difficulty accepting personal responsibility for what is happening to their health or illness. They find it hard to accept that their life choices are related to their experience of disease. They want professionals to find the right answer and "fix the disease."

Even though the atmosphere at the Kaslow Centers is very supportive and promotes the attitude that seriously ill persons can and will get better through informed personal action, such people find it hard to give up the "victim" role learned and rein- forced by the past. No one is *blamed* for being ill; that's not the point. It is simply pointed out that uninformed and unwise choices have been made. These can now become informed and wise choices based on new self-knowledge. These decisions will change the course of the disease.

It is a personal decision, not a treatment decision. This is at the root of success for most Kaslow patients. It is a delight for them to discover that their body *knows how to get well.*

LEARNING TO REBALANCE

Each person who participates in the Kaslow Medical Self-Care Program completes a Diet Survey (found in Chapter 8), experiences the nonprocessed carbohydrate test meal described in Chapter 3, undertakes a two-day distilled water fast, and proceeds through a series of tests of individual foods to assess body reaction to each.

These activities are designed as learning experiences. Each person discovers more about present eating habits, responses to and the effects of these habits, and the relationship between nutrition habits and feelings of illness or well-being.

Out of these activities emerges a three-stage self-awareness process: looking at what I am doing now and how it affects me, exploring alternative choices which may work better, and planning new habits that support my health.

Here are some of the activities and illustrations of how people change their views and habits:

The Surprise of Fasting

Prior to beginning the testing of individual foods for possible rejectivity, each patient fasts, drinking only distilled water for 48 hours. To the surprise of many, disease symptoms frequently disappear during this period and they may gain a general feeling of well-being toward the end of the fasting period. This certainly relates eating habits to disease. It also casts doubt on the advisability of trying to fix problems through intervention rather than getting out of the body's way and allowing it to heal itself. *When you do nothing and get better,* this is a strong signal that what you have been doing in the past is part of the problem.

As a result of this experience, many patients decide to fast for short periods on a regular basis. Many set aside one day a week to allow the body to relax and reestablish balance.

The Survey as a Mirror

Most people completing a diet survey have never stopped to make such a complete record of their eating patterns. Many are surprised by what they learn from this simple exercise. The types of food eaten, the frequency of eating each food, and the variety of foods (or lack of it) are quickly brought into focus. Habits or addictions are easily revealed.

Have you ever sat down and counted the number of soft drinks, candy bars, snack foods, and "goodies" you consume in a week? Many patients, when interviewed, find that they have not even listed these items, thinking they were unimportant since they were not "meals." Of course, everything we take into our bodies must be dealt with by our bodies in some way.

Thus, the survey acts like a mirror, reflecting back to each person details not previously seen. Frequently, this awareness alone triggers change in unwanted habits.

Realization of Limited Choices

There are thousands of plants and animal food sources in existence in our environment. As a result of cultural interests, the evolution of food production, and local growing conditions, only about 300 of these foods are generally available. To the surprise of most patients completing a survey, their habits include only 12 or fifteen foods. Convenience when shopping, habit, preparation patterns, and family history have all served to compress the available choices over time until very few foods are brought into the home and prepared for meals.

Like most Americans, Kaslow patients buy their foods in supermarkets. Easy-to-prepare packaged foods have gradually eased out fresh foods, which may take more time to clean, may require special recipes, or may spoil in the refrigerator. These tendencies toward the use of easy-to-prepare foods are especially pronounced among surveyed patients who live alone or have some difficulty getting out to shop.

The recognition that narrow choices of foods can lead to a greater possibility of rejectivity and illness fosters an interest in exploration of new foods. Lists of foods (to be found in Chapter 8) give clues and suggestions for wider variety.

Sensitivity and Body-Knowledge

During the nonprocessed carbohydrate test and the one-at-a-time food testing for rejectivity, each patient acquires perhaps for the first time a new level of sensitivity, relating food choices to moods, illness symptoms, and swings from health to dysfunction. This sensitivity is increased throughout the food-testing period. Eventually, individuals become distinctly aware of foods they can enjoy, foods that do not function properly in the body, and their needs for essential food materials and elements.

As with our laboratory animal friends mentioned earlier, there is no objective explanation for the high level of awareness one can develop about food selections related to needs. Just walking along the aisle in the store, a person will see a food that "feels right" for a meal planned that day. Patients learn to trust this inner sense of what they need in the context of a broad plan of variety.

WHAT IS GOOD FOOD?

If square meals from the basic four and fat-fried fast-foods are not good food, then how do we define good food?

Good food is natural. The continuing trend in the American agribusiness to stimulate ever-greater production per acre through intensive use of chemical fertilizers, herbicides (to kill weeds), and pesticides is destined to become an issue similar in magnitude to the current national debate about nuclear energy. Farm products and the ground water in farm areas are becoming increasingly contaminated by life-altering chemicals used to kill weeds and insects. In addition, the essential mineral content of foods is diminishing as greater amounts of chemical fertilizers are used instead of organic fertilizers.

If you can find stores in your area that feature natural or organic foods, we highly recommend that you patronize them rather than the large supermarket chains. Unfortunately, not everyone will be able to do this. An alternative is to plant a garden. If you enjoy gardening, this will offer you an excellent alternative to commercially produced foods.

If you continue to purchase supermarket foods, we recommend a daily supplement of a significant multiplex vitamin and an intake of at least 500–1000 mg. of vitamin C to give your body added capacity to breakdown and use these foods.

Good food is not refined or processed. Manufactured foods almost invariably involve the removal of several essential vitamin and mineral components from the harvested food. Even though the processed food may be "enriched" in the manufacturing process, only some of the essential elements of the original food are added back in. Also, almost all processed foods contain refined sugar and unwanted amounts of salt.

Good food does not include refined sugar. In our chapter on metabolic rejectivity, we described the long-term degenerating effect on the liver/pancreas system for metabolizing carbohydrates caused by overuse of simple carbohydrates. The rising incidence of hypoglycemic reaction and sugar diabetes is evidence of this overload. Historically, sugar was considered a preservative for fruits and vegetables and has only recently been so widely used as a "food." If you are interested in a well-written and entertaining account of the sociological history of sugar and its economic and political impact in America, we highly recommend *Sugar Blues*, a delightful book by William Dufty.

Good food is fresh. Fresh produce, fish, chicken, etc. deliver greater nutritional value than processed or preserved foods —the closer to picking or butchering the better. If you have stores available which offer fresh foods, we recommend that you make a special effort to obtain them.

Good food is light. Heavy, square meals are much more than is required for anyone other than a person who does hard

physical labor most of the day. Even if you are a regular exer-
ciser, three big meals a day in the American tradition is too much
food. Salads, fresh vegetables, eggs, fish, chicken, and other light
foods have all the nutritional elements your body needs. Eat
lightly. Your body will accommodate to the smaller intake and
you will feel better.

Good food is not overcooked.   In fact, most fresh vegetables
are best eaten raw. Slightly steamed vegetables and roasted or
broiled meats are preferable to boiled and fried foods. If you do
boil vegetables or cook them covered with water, save the water
for soup stock, as it is rich in the vitamins and minerals from
the vegetables. Frying breaks down many of the nutritionally
valuable components of foods and makes them more difficult to
digest.

Good food is variety.   As you know by now, food rejectivity is one of the major risks of persons experiencing health
problems. Rejectivity is a greater risk if your food choices are
limited to just a few foods eaten repeatedly. Vary your diet from
day to day and week to week. Try new foods. The risk of problems with rejectivity will diminish and you will also gain the
benefit of a more balanced intake from a variety of nutritional
elements from various foods.

Good food is enjoyed in an appropriate setting.   Recently,
America has developed the habit of eating on the run. Gulping
down a sandwich or hamburger while standing at an elevated
counter sets up conflicting activities in the body. Finding time
and an appropriate setting to savor food and appreciate its
nourishment can actually change the chemistry of digestion and
increase the value of the food to your body's requirement for
nourishment.

Good food is food your body can use.   Foods your body
rejects will deliver no nutritional value to you at all. They will
be passed through unmetabolized, and on the way will have
caused a great deal of stress and upset. Discovering and eliminating those foods to which you are not tolerant is a major step
toward significant improvement in your nutrition.

THE ROLE OF VITAMINS
IN SELF-REGULATION

Nutrition has traditionally been seen as the use of foods for the body's energy action and for cell and structure building and maintenance. As we have commented before, we see a very important third function: supply of the components for the self-regulation system in the body. Science is just beginning to gain insight into the key role vitamins, especially vitamin C, play in the process of self-regulation.

Dr. Constance R. Spittle of Pinderfields General Hospital in Wakefield, England, was puzzled by rapidly rising cholesterol levels in the blood of atherosclerotic patients following large doses of vitamin C. According to traditional measures, patients with rapidly rising cholesterol levels should have experienced pain, discomfort, and even crisis. Instead, these patients *improved quickly.* Her hypothesis was that the vitamin C somehow acted as a cleanser, picking up stored cholesterol from the arterial walls and transporting it out through the liver. In this view, the additional cholesterol in the blood was being carried out of the system, rather than accumulating. Hence, pressure in the arterial walls was relieved, diminishing the symptoms of cardiovascular distress.

Our hypothesis is somewhat different. We would say that the patient's cholesterol regulation system had been somehow distorted, perhaps by insufficient vitamin C. Therefore, when the person ate foods containing cholesterol, the internal regulation system for assessing needs for this substance failed to recognize the accumulation of an excess. The cholesterol continued to accumulate.

The internal cholesterol regulator apparently uses vitamin C as an integral part of its function. When inadequate vitamin C is available, the regulator malfunctions. When large doses of vitamin C were taken, an adequate supply was made available. The regulator, like the receptor cells we spoke of in the insulin/ glucose interaction and the appetite monitor in the glycerol/ overweight examples, was able to function once this barrier was overcome. The body immediately recognized excess cholesterol and began to remove it through the liver in normal fashion, and the patient's condition improved.

Another very different example of regulator involvement of vitamins has been reported relating vitamin C to effective function of the immune system in response to infection.

Gary Thurman and Allan Goldstein of George Washington University conducted tests exposing two groups of guinea pigs to the tuberculosis bacterium. One group was assured of adequate vitamin C, the other was deprived of vitamin C. The animals were then tested for the efficiency of their immune responses to the bacterium and for their ability to create antibodies against a foreign substance, in this case sheep blood cells.

Tissue levels of vitamin C in the deprived guinea pigs fell within three weeks, their immune responses became very depressed, and twice as many of the deprived animals collapsed and died in comparison to the supplied animals. These findings substantiate evidence that the immune system depends on an adequate supply of vitamin C to fight infections and develop adequate antibodies.

Science is just beginning to explore these intricate relationships. Linus Pauling has led the way in the investigation of the role of vitamins in the prevention and amelioration of all disease. However, much of the emphasis, as it is still presently perceived incorrectly, is on how to use vitamins to fix disease.

Our perspective, again, is that nutritional elements, especially vitamins, play a key role in the natural self-regulation of the body. This simplifies the matter greatly. Instead of seeking the exact formula for the role each vitamin may play in each disease or malfunction, all we need to do is see that the body receives a reasonable amount of every needed element, including vitamins, and the body will handle the problem on its own. It may be a long time before science discovers all these intricate relationships within the body. In the meantime, the body knows how to manage itself if it has the elements it needs and the distorting factors on self-regulation are recognized, reduced or eliminated.

THE VITAMINS AND MINERALS

Table 5.2 lists the vitamins, minerals, and trace elements which are significant to the health of the body. It is excerpted from a wall chart available from Elixir Enterprises, P.O. Box 14216,

Lansing, Michigan 49804. Our list shows the biological function of each element, the symptoms of deficiency, and factors which deplete the element from the body. Should you be experiencing considerable stress, or any of the depleting factors listed on our earlier chart, you may want to include vitamin and mineral supplements in your food program to make up for these factors.

Following this table we have listed some principal food sources of each of these elements in Table 5.3. For a more complete assessment of the elements in many foods, we highly recommend Dr. Roger Williams's book, *The Wonderful World Within You*, especially Chapter 15, "How to Choose Your Own Nourishment."

Using our tables or Dr. Williams's book, anyone can plan a variety of meals including many different foods that naturally supply all the elements the body needs. In the Chapter 8 workbook, you can learn to test foods to determine your acceptance or nontolerance of them. During that process, you will begin to create Chinese-style meals consisting of small portions of several foods already "accepted" by your body. The eventual outcome of your food testing and planning process will be a diet of meals, light in style, consisting of a wide variety of foods. Through such a program, your body should get all the nutrient value it needs.

Although the Kaslow Program emphasizes freedom from chronic disease through nutrition it also recognizes that many patients are doubtful about their ability to change the course of their disease. In the next chapter we present a scenario that has helped others step away from the position of "no hope" that medicine has placed them in once their "incurable" chronic disease has been diagnosed.

Table 5.2: VITAMINS, MINERALS, AND TRACE ELEMENTS

VITAMIN/MINERAL CHEMICAL PROPERTIES (STABILITY)	BIOLOGICAL FUNCTION	DEFICIENCY SYMPTOMS	DEPLETING FACTORS
A CAROTENE: PREFORMED A fat soluble; stable to heat; unstable to air; destroyed by ultra-violet	Essential for growth of young; increases resistance to urinary and respiratory infection; lactation and reproduction; night vision (visual purple); proper appetite and digestion; skin health	Allergies; brittle hair and dry skin; ear abscesses; fatigue; night blindness; poor appetite; poor digestion and tooth formation; retarded growth; sinus problems; sterility	Mineral oil; cortisone and other drugs; excess alcohol and iron consumption; polyunsaturated fats taken without anti-oxident; coffee; smoking; pollution; vitamin D deficiency
B COMPLEX B1 THIAMINE water soluble, unstable to ultra-violet; destroyed by boiling in acidic solution, heat	Absorption and digestion; appetite; blood building; carbohydrate metabolism; corrects and prevents beriberi; learning ability; promotes growth, resistance to infection and proper nerve function	Beriberi; fatigue; intestinal disorders; irritability; nerve degeneration; numbness of hands and feet; poor lactation and appetite; shortness of breath; slow heart beat; ulcers; weakness	Alcohol; antibiotics; birth control pills; coffee; diuretics; diarrhea; excess sugar; fever; raw clams and oysters; stress; surgery
B2 RIBOFLAVIN; VITAMIN G water soluble; stable to air, heat; unstable to visible light, u.v.; destroyed by alkalies	Antibody and red blood cell formation; aids iron assimilation and protein metabolism; healthy skin and digestive tract; prolongs life; promotes growth and general health; vision	Cataracts; digestive disturbances; hair loss; impaired lactation; lack of stamina; pellagra; reduced tissue respiration; retarded growth; tongue ulceration; weight loss	Alcohol; birth control pills; coffee; excessive sugar; tobacco—need increases in proportion to muscular work
B3 NIACIN water soluble; stable to heat; light air, acid and alkali	Circulation; hormone (sex) production; growth; hydrochloric acid production; main-	Appetite loss; canker sores; depression; fatigue; halitosis; headache; indigestion; insom-	Alcohol; antibiotics; birth control pills; coffee; corn; excessive sugar and starches;

Elixir Enterprises (P.O. Box 14216, Lansing, Michigan 49804), reprinted with permission.

Table 5.2, cont.

VITAMIN/MINERAL CHEMICAL PROPERTIES (STABILITY)	BIOLOGICAL FUNCTION	DEFICIENCY SYMPTOMS	DEPLETING FACTORS
	tenance of nervous system; metabolism; reduces cholesterol level; respiration	nia; muscular weakness; nausea; nerve disorders; skin problems	growth periods; illness; physical labor; tissue trauma
B5 PANTOTHENIC ACID water soluble; unstable to heat; destroyed by acid & alkali (vinegar—baking soda)	Antibody formation; carbohydrate metabolism; growth stimulation; healthy skin and nerves; maintains blood sugar level; stimulates adrenals; vitamin utilization	Adrenal exhaustion; depression; diarrhea; hair loss; hypoglycemia; intestinal disorders; kidney problems; nerve disorders; premature aging; skin disorders	Alcohol; coffee; insecticide; sleeping pills; stress
B6 PYRIDOXINE water soluble; stable in heat; unstable in light	Antibody formation; controls level of magnesium in blood and tissues; digestion; maintains sodium/potassium balance; cholesterol levels; metabolism of fats	Acne; anemia; arthritis; behavioral changes; convulsion in infants; dizziness; hair loss; irritability; learning disabilities; swelling; weakness	Aging; alcohol; birth control pills; heart attack; insecticide; radiation exposure; sleeping pills; tobacco
B12 CYANOCOBALAMIN water soluble	Appetite; blood cell formation; cell longevity; normal metabolism of nerve tissue: protein, fat and carbohydrate metabolism; utilization of iron	Menstrual disturbances; nervousness; soreness and weakness in extremities; symptoms of schizophrenia; walking and speaking difficulties	Aging; alcohol; coffee; insecticide; iron, calcium and B6 deficiency; laxatives; sleeping pills; tobacco
B15 PANGAMIC ACID water soluble	Cell oxidation and respiration; stimulates glucose, fat, protein metabolism, glandular and nervous system	Diminished oxidation of cells; glandular and nervous disorders; heart disease	Alcohol; birth control pills; coffee; insecticide; sleeping pills

CHEMICAL PROPERTIES (STABILITY	BIOLOGICAL FUNCTION	DEFIENCY SYMPTOMS	DEPLETING FACTORS
BIOTIN, VITAMIN H water soluble; stable to heat; inactivated by oxidation; synthesized by intestinal bacteria	Growth, lipid synthesis in liver; metabolism of carbohydrates; fats, protein; vitamin B utilization	Disturbed nervous system; dry skin; eczema; grayish skin; hair loss; insomnia; impaired fat formation; irregular heart beat; mental depression; muscular pain; physical weakness	Alcohol; birth control pills; coffee; insecticide: raw egg white (Avidin); sleeping pills
CHOLINE water soluble	Health of liver, kidney and nervous tissue; prevents gall stones; with inositol is basic constituent of lecithin; utilization of fats	Bleeding ulcers; fatty deposits in liver; growth problems; heart trouble; high blood pressure; kidney blockage	Alcohol; birth control pills; coffee; excess sugar; insecticide; sleeping pills
FOLIC ACID water soluble; destroyed by heat and light	Aids liver performance; appetite; cell reproduction; growth; HCL production; protein metabolism; red blood cell formation	Anemia; digestive disturbances; graying hair; mental illness; poor growth; tongue inflammation	Alcohol; antacids; birth control pills; coffee; laxatives; stress; sulfa drugs (Aminoperin, Streptomycin); tobacco
INOSITOL water soluble	Brain cell nutrition; fat metabolism; growth and survival of cells in bone marrow, eye and intestines; hair health; lecithin formation; reduces blood cholesterol; protects liver, kidney and heart	Constipation; eczema: eye abnormalities; hair loss; high blood cholesterol	Alcohol; birth control pills; coffee; insecticide; sleeping pills

Table 5.2, cont.

VITAMIN/MINERAL CHEMICAL PROPERTIES (STABILITY)	BIOLOGICAL FUNCTION	DEFICIENCY SYMPTOMS	DEPLETING FACTORS
PARA AMINOBENZOIC ACID (PABA) water soluble	Blood cell formation; hair pigment; stimulates intestinal bacteria to form folic acid; protein metabolism; sunscreen	Constipation; depression; digestive disturbances; fatigue; gray hair; headache; irritability; nervousness	Alcohol; birth control pills; coffee; insecticide; sleeping pills; sulfa drugs
C ASCORBIC ACID water soluble; stable to heat; destroyed by oxygen, u.v., copper and iron cooking vessels, pasteurization, canning, insecticide	Appetite; blood vessel health; calcium diffusion; prevents vitamin oxidation; promotes growth and healing; proper bone and tooth formation; protects heart; raises resistance to infection; red blood cell formation	Anemia; bleeding gums; bruise easily; capillary ruptures; dental caries; headache; impaired adrenal function; lowered resistance to infection; pernicious anemia; scurvy; ulcers	Antibiotics; anxiety; aspirin; burns; cortisone; fatigue; high fever; inhalation of DDT or petroleum fumes; stress; sulfa drugs, tobacco; water (excess)
D CALCIFEROL fat soluble; stable to light, heat and air	Absorption and metabolism of calcium and phosphorus; clotting; heart action; proper gland and nerve function; tooth and bone formation; skin respiration	Constipation; dental caries; insomnia; lack of stamina; muscular weakness; myopia; nervousness; tetany	Mineral oil
E TOCOPHEROL stable to visible light, heat, acid and alkali; destroyed by u.v. light; rancid fats reduce its potency	Blood flow to heart; fertility; lung protection; male potency; prevents toxemia of pregnancy; pituitary regulation; reduces blood cholesterol; retards aging	Brittle and falling hair; deficient lactation; gastro-intestinal disease; impotency; miscarriage; sterility	Air pollution; birth control pills; chlorine; illness; iron; mineral oil; rancid fats and oils
F UNSATURATED FATTY ACIDS easily destroyed when exposed to air, may become rancid	Assimilates phosphorus; growth; glandular activity; organ respiration; reduces	Acne; allergies; baldness; brittle nails; circulation and kidney disorders; dandruff; diarrhea;	Radiation; X rays

VITAMIN/MINERAL CHEMICAL PROPERTIES (STABILITY)	BIOLOGICAL FUNCTION	DEFICIENCY SYMPTOMS	DEPLETING FACTORS
	blood cholesterol; regulates rate of blood coagulation; vitamin A production	eczema; gall stones; heart and skin disorders; hot weather distress; nail problems; under-weight; varicose veins	Air pollution: antibiotics (excessive); aspirin; colitis; diarrhea; frozen foods; mineral oil; radiation; rancid fats; sprue; X rays
K MENADIONE fat soluble	Blood clotting (prevents hemorrhage); vital for normal liver function; vitality and longevity factor	Cellular disease; diarrhea; hemorrhaging; increased clotting time; miscarriage: nose bleeds	Same as C
P BIOFLAVONOIDS water soluble; occurs with vitamin C showing similar chemical properties	Alters permeability of capillaries; increases resistance to colds and flu; maintains healthy connective tissue and blood vessel walls; proper absorption of vitamin C; strengthens capillary walls	Same as C	
CALCIUM	Aids general mineral and vitamin metabolism; bone/tooth formation; clotting; nerve and muscle response; promotes normal behavior and mental alertness; proper heart actions; pH regulation, reduces fatigue	Bone malformation; cramps; heart palpitations; joint pain; impaired growth; insomnia; nervousness; numbness in extremities	Aging; excessive stress; sugars; inactivity; large amounts of phytic acid (grain, cereals)
COPPER	Assists hemoglobin and red	Anemia; edema; general weak-	High zinc intake

Table 5.2, cont.

VITAMIN/MINERAL CHEMICAL PROPERTIES (STABILITY)	BIOLOGICAL FUNCTION	DEFICIENCY SYMPTOMS	DEPLETING FACTORS
	blood cell formation; healing; oxidation of vitamin C; present in metabolic enzymes; protein metabolism; proper bone formation; RNA synthesis; skin and hair pigmentation; synthesis of phospholipids	ness; impaired respiration; skin sores	
IODINE	Aids nutritive process; balances general glandular system; color and texture of hair; energy production; excess fat metabolism; promotes growth and development; proper thyroid function; stimulates circulatory system	Cretinism; dry hair; goiter; hardening of arteries; heart palpitations; irritability; obesity; polio; slowed mental reaction; sluggish metabolism; rapid pulse	Deficiency may be caused by certain compounds in raw cabbage and nuts
IRON	Absorbs and carries oxygen as a component of hemoglobin; increases resistance to stress and disease; necessary for health of all cells	Breathing difficulties; brittle nails; constipation; iron deficiency anemia (pale skin and abnormal fatigue)	Coffee; excess phosphorus, zinc; high cellulose intake; lack of HCL; rapid intestinal movement
MAGNESIUM	Aids in elimination of foreign matter and waste; albumen formation; builds cells particularly of lung and nervous tissue; calcium and vitamin C metabolism; constituent of muscle;	Apprehensiveness; brain and body exhaustion; confusion; disorientation; glandular disturbances; irritability; muscle twitch; poor circulation and complexion; tremors	Diarrhea; diuretics; excess alcohol, protein consumption; high blood cholesterol

VITAMIN/MINERAL CHEMICAL PROPERTIES (STABILITY)	BIOLOGICAL FUNCTION	DEFICIENCY SYMPTOMS	DEPLETING FACTORS
	gives strength and firmness to bone and teeth; regulates blood pH		
PHOSPHORUS	Active transport; bone and tooth formation; kidney function; metabolism of fats, carbohydrates and protein; nerve transmission; nucleoprotein formation; regulates blood pH; skeletal growth; stimulates muscle contractions	Appetite loss; irregular breathing; mental and physical fatigue; nervous disorders; weight loss or overweight	Excessive aluminum, iron, magnesium and white sugar intake; antacids; high-fat diet
POTASSIUM	Assists kidney function; balances acids; counterbalances Na action; gives pliancy to muscular tissue; glycogen formation; maintains proper fluid balance; neuromuscular contraction; normal growth	Acne; constipation; dry skin; general weakness; impairment of neuromuscular function; insomnia; nervous disorders; poor reflexes; slow irregular heart beat; thirst	Alcohol; aldosterone; coffee; cortisone; diuretics; excessive salt and sugar; laxatives; prolonged diarrhea, sweating; stress
SODIUM	Elimination of CO_2; formation of digestive juices; saliva, bile, pancreatic juices; keeps blood minerals soluble; muscle con-	Appetite loss; gas; impaired fat conversion; muscle shrinkage; vomiting; weight loss	Diarrhea; diuretics; lack of chlorine or potassium; perspiration; vomiting

Table 5.2, cont.

VITAMIN/MINERAL CHEMICAL PROPERTIES (STABILITY)	BIOLOGICAL FUNCTION	DEFICIENCY SYMPTOMS	DEPLETING FACTORS
	traction: nerve impulses; regulates water balance and blood pH		
SULPHUR	Antiseptic and cleansing effect on alimentary tract; constituent of hemoglobin; keeps hair glossy and complexion clear; maintains body resistance; maintains and matures cells; normalizes heart action; prevents toxic accumulation; purifies blood; stimulates bile secretion	Brittle nails; splitting hair	Unknown
ZINC	Alcohol breakdown; B1; carbohydrate assimilation: healing burns and wounds; maintenance of healthy tissue; normal prostrate function; phosphorus and protein metabolism; reproductive organ growth and development	Decreased alertness; delayed sexual maturity; fatigue; loss of taste; prolong healing; retarded growth; sterility	Alcohol; high calcium and phytic acid (grains) intake; lack of phosphorus

Table 5.3:   PRINCIPAL FOOD SOURCES OF
VITAMINS, MINERALS, AND TRACE ELEMENTS

Vitamin A (Carotene)—Broccoli, carrots, kale, sweet potatoes, beef
liver, calf liver, chicken liver

Vitamin B1 (Thiamine)—Lima beans, peas, soybeans, millet, wheat
germ, peanuts, sunflower seeds

Vitamin B2 (Riboflavin)—Liver and kidney

Vitamin B3 (Niacin)—Organ meats, peanuts, rhubarb, halibut, mackerel,
some in peas, soybeans, and grains

Vitamin B5 (Pantothenic Acid)—Organ meats, mushrooms, peanuts,
whole grains

Vitamin B6 (Pyridoxine)—Rice, peas, salmon, organ meats, prunes

Vitamin B12 (Cyanocobalamin)—Liver, tuna, cheese, eggs

Vitamin B15 (Pangamic Acid)—Brewer's Yeast, brown rice, organ meats,
sesame, sunflower and pumpkin seeds, wheat germ, whole grains

Vitamin C (Ascorbic Acid)—Broccoli, kale, sweet peppers, cantaloupe,
oranges, strawberries

Vitamin D (Calciferol)—Salmon, milk, eggs, sunlight

Vitamin E (Tocopherol)—Wheat germ, safflower oil, peanuts, vegetable
oil

Vitamin F (Unsaturated Fatty Acids)—Corn, safflower, soy and wheat
germ oil, sunflower seeds

Vitamin H (Biotin)—Beef liver, soy beans, mung sprouts, brewer's yeast

Vitamin K (Menadione)—Spinach, brussel sprouts, soybeans

Vitamin P (Bioflavonoids)—Currants, buckwheat, cherries, grapes,
grapefruit, lemons, plums (ten times as much in the fruit as in juices)

Calcium—Green vegetables, egg yolk, dairy foods, sardines, salmon,
shellfish, broccoli, kale, soybeans

Copper—Sweet potatoes, lima beans, citrus fruits, beef liver, pork,
mushrooms, mackerel, whole rye, asparagus, almonds, avocado,
cabbage, chicken, beef, kale, lobster, halibut, grapes, oats, shellfish,
spinach, turkey, walnuts, wheat, eggs, apples, bananas, corn, carrots

Iodine—Cod liver oil, iodized salt, mushrooms

Table 5.3, cont.

Iron—Liver sausage, all legumes, dried beans, soy beans, lean meat, egg yolk, green leafy vegetables, whole grains, liver, peaches, organ meats, shellfish, other sea foods

Magnesium—Raw tomatoes, lima beans, raw carrots, roast poultry, roasted nuts, whole wheat, boiled spinach, citrus fruits, baked beans, fresh peas, codfish, brown rice, oats, peaches, peanuts, potatoes, soy flour, barley, corn

Manganese—Whole rye, whole wheat, sweet potatoes, snap beans, whole corn, liver, oats, spinach, bananas, beets, lettuce, kale, dried beans

Phosphorus—Pumpkin seeds, brazil nuts, wheat germ, beef liver, all protein rich foods such as eggs, fish and meat

Potassium—Potatoes, especially the skin, bananas, plus small amounts in many foods

Sodium—Cheeses, greens, milk, seafood, salt in most prepared or canned foods (use of much table salt discouraged)

Sulphur—Protein rich foods, beans, bran, brussels sprouts, cabbage, cauliflower, cheese, shellfish

Zinc—Protein rich foods, beans, bran, brussels sprouts, brewer's yeast, greens, liver, pumpkin seeds

6

MOVING FROM HELPLESSNESS TO ACTION

HELEN L., 56, ARRIVED AT THE KASLOW CENTER LOOKING like a woman in her 70s or 80s. She moved with great difficulty and needed a cane. Her hands and feet were swollen and in pain. Her teeth and gums were so sensitive that she could hardly brush her teeth.

Helen was suffering from rheumatoid arthritis. She felt that she was being punished by her body and was deeply depressed. She took two different pain medications each day, but nothing her physicians had suggested seemed to relieve her pain or offer her promise of a more comfortable and productive future. Helen felt she was a helpless victim of the disease and had lost control of the forces that directed her life.

Louise R., 60, began her journey as a medical patient at age 16. Feeling low in energy and suffering from gas and indigestion, she was one of the first patients to be treated a number of years ago with cortisone. She can no longer remember exactly what purpose the cortisone was to serve, but it initiated a life dependent on drugs and the medical system.

When she was 28, physicians discovered that her fertility had been affected by the long-term use of cortisone and a new round of drugs followed. She found herself in a continuing spiral of more and different drugs and growing dependency on doctors. Antispasmodic medications for a hernia, antinausea medications three times a day for indigestion, and frequent antibiotics for flu and respiratory difficulties had come to dominate her daily routine. Louise also could not control her weight.

She began to feel she was at the mercy of her many medical problems. Her life was molded around her role as a relatively helpless medical patient, trying to manage her problems in a complex routine of seemingly unrelated treatments and drugs.

Both these cases are fairly typical of the repeating pattern of helplessness and despair among people who seek traditional medical care for chronic problems. Patients feel victimized by their diseases, dependent on professionals who are sometimes indifferent to their distress, and completely lacking in control over any of the factors that will determine their futures.

Helen gained some insights at the Kaslow Center. She had grown to expect pain and failure from her body without knowing the cause. She quickly learned that eating sweets and highly sugared processed foods aggravated the pains and dysfunctions. She eliminated these foods from her diet and her body began to respond.

Helen had given up on her natural sense of balance and her expectation that her hands and fingers would ever again do what she wanted them to do. Learning to walk in a swimming pool where her fear of falling was diminished, she began to regain her sense of balance. Small tasks, such as buttoning buttons and picking up toothpicks, restored her confidence in the use of her hands and fingers, reversing the negative attitudes she had held about the abilities of her body.

Recently Helen wrote a letter to the Kaslow staff happily relating a trip to the dentist during which her teeth were cleaned without pain. She is visiting restaurants without the fear that her use of silverware will be clumsy or that she might knock over a water glass. Helen is rebuilding her confidence and sense of control over her own life. She can walk without pain and has given up all medication.

Louise came to the Kaslow Center in late 1977. She expressed surprise that she was treated with dignity and that someone believed her problems were worthy of consideration. She learned through a stool analysis that her long-term use of cortisone had affected the natural enzyme production in her digestive system, interfering with her metabolization of foods (hence her low energy and nausea). Louise learned through personal Response Diet testing that fruits caused pounding of the heart, sweating, and shortness of breath. She eliminated these problem foods from her diet.

Louise took up walking and swimming to get a new sense of movement and flexibility. She no longer takes any medication and says, "I walk or swim a half hour each day and I feel great. I'm going to get my Ph.D. soon and start living again."

The Kaslow Program is a very different medical approach for Helen and Louise and for others suffering from long-term illness. The program focuses not on what is wrong and how the doctor can manipulate the problem, but instead on what individuals can do on their own to improve health, flexibility, and function.

The entire Kaslow staff, instead of treating diseases, supports patients with the attitude that they can and will get better as a result of their own initiative and action. Patients are assured that they have a way out of pain and illness and that their personal choices and perseverance can lead them to success.

Processes at the Kaslow Centers are designed to provide prompt and direct feedback so that patients can experience their own feelings, moods, and physical responses to the activities there. In the description of the Kaslow Program in Chapter 7, and in the workbook in Chapter 8, you discover these self-learning elements of the Kaslow Program.

Let's take a look at the old attitudes of helplessness most patients have learned, why they are so widely held, and their usual outcomes. Then, we can compare them to new attitudes that can be learned, why these seem to be successful, and the outcomes they have been shown to produce.

OLD ATTITUDES OF HELPLESSNESS

- My personal attitudes and actions are not necessarily important to, or involved in, the future of my health and/or disease condition.

- I am ill and need to be made well. My disease is an enemy that has attacked me and I must fight to overcome my condition.

- I am essentially ignorant about what is happening to me. Knowledge of the process of my disease and the steps to be taken to improve my condition are privileged information held by doctors.

- Therefore, I am helpless to act unless I can find the physician or clinic that can make me well.

- If I am unable to find someone who can make me well, I am doomed to a life of disability and failure.

These attitudes, which condemn a person to a position of powerlessness and inaction, have grown out of our country's history of fear of and lack of knowledge about how our bodies work. This fear and lack of knowledge has led to a denial of the malfunctioning body (seeing the disease as something other than a part of oneself), a position as victim of some malevolent natural force, and dependency on professionals who have the intricate know-how to manipulate natural forces within the body.

The Victim Position

In Chapter 2 we discussed at length our culture's view of nature as adversary. Our medical system has sought the identity of invading entities as the causes of all diseases and portrays patients as helpless victims of these entities. The relationship among food allergies, nutritional habits, stress, exercise, and disease has only recently been explored.

The victim position leads the sufferer of disease to separate the disease from the body and look at it as another entity. Until this entity can be removed, the patient is burdened with it.

The Kaslow position proposes that disease is a result of malfunction of self-regulation in the body. Since the patient can learn to identify those choices in life which lead to this malfunction and change them, he or she is no longer a helpless victim.

Professional Dependency

Information about self-care and the understanding of our bodies has not been generally available until recently. We have been taught to accept that this information is the exclusive province of the physician. Physicians say, "A little knowledge is a dangerous thing. People will be trying to treat their own problems with disastrous results."

Since we remain relatively ignorant of the functions of the body, we feel helpless and incompetent when illness develops. We take the problems to a physician whom we assume will be all-knowing. We literally transfer ownership of our bodies to the medical system.

The symptoms of our illnesses become separate from our person. "The headaches, my arthritis, the pain in my left foot" are now the property of the physician. He or she now owns the problem, may refer it to a specialist, who may then refer it to another specialist, until "they" decide what to do about it. The patient may gain little or no insight into what is being considered. Much of this process may occur with little thought to the emotional, social, or financial impact on the patient and family. The physician talks about owning a practice, which is essentially a list of patients. Patients tend to be thought of in terms of problems or symptoms, such as the gall bladder in room 112.

The physician's role is to manage the progression of the symptoms. This leaves the patient with the relatively helpless role of follower of instructions. This is called "patient compliance."

The Kaslow Premise is that ownership of the body must be returned to the patient so that he or she can begin to solve the problem at its source. The entire process at the Kaslow Centers is designed to be educational, offering each patient the skills and knowledge to identify the onset of difficulties, locate the factors that contribute to the problem, change the life situation to diminish the effect of those factors, and regain control over the future.

Lack of Knowledge

Our fears about illness, pain, and dysfunction are based on our lifetime of experience in a society that places little or no emphasis on self-understanding of health and body function.

America has perhaps the most comprehensive and widespread program of general public education ever undertaken. We go to school for 12, 16, or perhaps even more years to learn skills to function as productive adults. The most essential skill, *how to understand and care for our own health*, without which all the other skills and knowledge may become worthless, is forgotten in the rush to achieve material success. In a curriculum aimed at a broad base of knowledge, the most basic possession of each individual—the human body—is all but ignored. Even if a student should study biology or the natural sciences, the material is presented in the context of studying nature "out there," and little effort is made to relate the knowledge to self-function and health.

Take a survey of your local schools. It is unlikely that any of them, colleges included, offer a course entitled, "Basic Functions of the Human Body." If so, it is probably taken only by those studying health sciences or medicine. (It must be noted here that even medical schools rarely include in their curriculum a study of the role of nutrition in health and disease.)

There are advanced specialists in many fields of medicine and life science who attain significant knowledge of isolated aspects of biocellular activity, but cannot relate their research and education to personal life. Seeing this knowledge as relating to the world of nature "out there," which is somehow separate from human activity, these scientists regard serious chronic disease just like others in the society who have little or no knowledge of the body. As Pirsig said in *Zen and the Art of Motorcycle Maintenance*, reason has become separated from quality.

Our society's study of the human system has emphasized the labeling and analysis of each of the individual and minute parts and has failed to understand the true nature of the system of life in which each person functions.

In a nation of relatively well-educated people, trained to achieve economic success in the workplace, we might take a survey asking basic questions about body functions. Perhaps only the life scientists among us could answer such questons as:

- What are the major organ systems of the body and what is the function of each?

- What are the basic muscle systems of the body, how are

they interconnected, and how do you use them to perform day-to-day tasks?

- How does the body digest, assimilate, and metabolize foods?
- How does the body's immune system work?

At the Kaslow Centers, we find this lack of knowledge a significant barrier to rehabilitation of muscle flexibility and body movement. The patient is encouraged to learn about body function and develop a working knowledge of how each body movement is achieved through muscle action. This greater awareness alone is frequently a major step toward improved function.

THE PATHWAY TO HELPLESSNESS

Pain, distress, and dysfunction are signals from the body that a problem needs our attention. In our opening chapter, we related Linda Dunlap's story describing the episodes of dizziness, blurring of vision, and loss of balance she experienced. When Linda first encountered these episodes, she tried to ignore them and hoped they would go away on their own. Even though she was a nurse and had the advantage of knowledge many might not enjoy, she neither sought medical care nor thought there were actions she might take on her own to explore the problem.

Her resistance to seeking some sort of resolution to her problem is fairly typical of many who first experience pain, distress, and dysfunction in the body. This lack of self-knowledge creates a deep fear, first that we may have a dread disease, and second that we may have to undergo highly stressful and unpleasant interactions with the professional medical system.

The Fear of Knowing

This fear is the *fear of knowing*, which overtakes many who first begin to experience the onset of serious illness. Central to this fear is the possibility of having a dread disease involving more pain, protracted and painful treatments, disruption of life, and extended and costly medical care. The pain and dysfunction may represent serious illness, hence may cost us our job, our functional ability, our future, and there may even be a threat of death. Added to the fear are earlier memories of long waits in impersonal medical waiting rooms, the pain and humiliation of diagnostic examinations for other, earlier problems, the feelings of loss of personal integrity and dignity in medical settings, and panic at the thought of hospitalization and separation from family and those who care.

No one wants to learn he or she has an incurable disease. It is common to fear the complete rejection associated with the crippled, maimed, or incurably diseased. In Linda Dunlap's case, this fear was actually realized when her diagnosis of multiple sclerosis was finally announced and she was rejected and sent home by her physician with the admonition that nothing could be done.

In a case study examined in a brochure from the Muscular Dystrophy Association, the patient described a scene in a physician's office. The doctor asked him if his wife or a family member had accompanied him. His wife was in the waiting room and was invited in. The doctor then announced *to her* that her husband had muscular dystrophy and would slowly die a painful death. *The doctor never spoke another word directly to the patient.* As soon as the diagnosis of an incurable illness was confirmed, this patient ceased to exist as a competent person in the eyes of the medical system. Intuitively, we all fear being placed in that untenable position and will avoid the possibility as long as we can.

Patients become familiar, either through personal experience or from stories told by friends and relatives, with the loss of control experienced by individuals interacting with the "medical system." Painful diagnostic tests, separation from loved ones, anxiety-producing waiting rooms, and busy and indifferent personnel all make up the frequently repeated stories of "my operation" or "my visit to the clinic." Anyone who has heard these tales or had personal experience will consciously or unconsciously avoid interaction with the system in the future.

In addition, many people are learning that treatments for serious illnesses are equal to, if not more serious than, the pains and discomforts of the disease itself. A cortisone shot to relieve pain in an arthritic joint, although it may hold some promise of eventual relief, is a dreaded and painful experience. Therefore, people will delay confirming that they have arthritis to avoid the possibility of painful treatment.

Physicians may resort to "threats of dire consequences" to induce people to come in for early discovery of dread diseases; "If you don't find it early, it may kill you." Since fear of having the disease is one of the principal factors delaying examination, use of these strategies is completely counterproductive.

Dr. Patricia Kelly at the University of California Medical Center in San Francisco is conducting a study on breast self-examination which illustrates this point. Dr. Kelly reports that the recent great rush of information about breast cancer, especially mastectomy, has confused and frightened many women. Women fear cancer most as a disease. However, they fear the impersonal, imposing, and essentially male-dominated medical system as well. Many who have come to Dr. Kelly's research interviews reveal that their anxiety about the present medical model of practice is the central problem. Her program offers a nonthreatening way for these women to find out something about their anxieties *without having to see a physician or enter the medical system.* Dr. Kelly reports that fear of loss of control over their lives and their bodies has definitely prevented many women from seeking medical advice.

Some women who come to Dr. Kelly's program represent another pole. She discovers that they have had as many as six medical exams within the last year! They are obsessed with the fear of cancer and detailed these concerns to Dr. Kelly and her staff. This is a clear example of the next step on the pathway to helplessness: the fear of *not knowing.*

The Fear of Not Knowing

If pain, distress, or dysfunction persist and begin to interfere seriously with life patterns, the person eventually reaches a point at which he or she decides he/she must find out what is happening. Distress reaches the stage where *not knowing* creates a greater fear of the future than the threat of discovering the truth.

At this point, the patient will endure some of the indignities and costs of seeking medical care to obtain anxiety-reducing information about the problem. In Linda Dunlap's case, she tried desperately to find out what was happening to her as her symptoms increased in frequency and severity. Not knowing what was going on in her body created a greater sense of loss of control than she had feared might result from interacting with the medical system.

Part of us is afraid of what we will find out from medical professionals, but another part of us eventually becomes even more afraid of the uncertainty of not knowing.

The human being is essentially a self-knowing, self-directed creature. We seek to know and understand what is going on within us and around us and have great difficulty with an uncertain future. When we do not know, we seek a way to find out. In the case of illness, we have been taught that information about our bodies is solely the province of medical practitioners, so we must go to them for answers.

Traditional Medical Options

Once treatment is sought, there are three general possibilities for the course of action that will follow:

1. An early diagnosis will be obtained for some infectious or medically understood problem for which there is a reasonable and effective course of treatment. In this case, the problem is more or less resolved, the anxiety and fear disappear, and the patient improves.

2. There will be a protracted period of anxiety, expense, life disruption, and tests, without any satisfactory diagnosis of the problem or effective suggestions for a course of treatment. This may lead to a long-term dependency on the medical system, but eventually may also lead to resolution of the problem if some diagnosis is finally reached which suggests a workable course of treatment.

3. An "incurable" disease will be diagnosed. This will inevitably lead to a protracted series of treatments, whose sole purpose is to delay or ameliorate the effects of this disease, or to a "sentence" of disability—there is nothing to be done except to go home and live with the fact of eventual collapse and death.

To further clarify, Table 6.1 presents the four steps in the pathway to helplessness. The predictable destination for each traditional option is also indicated.

As long as the medical community continues to look on chronic and degenerative disease from the outdated perspective of an "invading-entity" infectious-type disease, more and more people are likely to end up in the helplessness and despair categories.

More and more money and effort is being put into extensive diagnostic procedures as doctors try to pin down all the minute cellular events in a person's body in the search for an exact description of a disease. Many patients coming to the Kaslow Centers have spent thousands of dollars on specialists and tests. The money was not spent on treatments to alleviate the disease, but on *diagnosis*, which failed to reveal a productive course of action.

Another possible road on the pathway to helplessness is a patient's life that revolves around medical care, symptoms, doctor's visits, and medications. Exhibiting a number of supposedly unrelated symptoms, this unhappy patient may be seeing two, three, or more physicians, each a specialist in one symptom.

One patient who came to the Kaslow Center was taking eight different medications. On examination, it became apparent that each drug had been added to the patient's routine in response to the side effects from the previous one. It's a familiar story. A patient goes to a physician seeking relief from headaches. A pain medication is prescribed. Soon thereafter, the patient returns complaining of indigestion. Another medication is prescribed to calm the upset stomach. The patient then begins to experience cramps and irregularity in her menstrual periods. She visits her gynecologist who prescribes a third medication without any knowledge of the sequence of events of the first two. This pattern of individual prescriptions continues through the occurrence of additional symptoms. None of the doctors ever considers that the patient's body *may simply be reeling under this massive effort to manipulate its internal processes.* The pyramid of side effects may finally dominate the person's life.

Through lack of coordination of the medical program, through diagnosis of "incurable" diseases, or through long-term

Table 6.1: STEPS ON THE PATHWAY TO HELPLESSNESS

1. ONSET OF PROBLEM	2. THE FEAR OF KNOWING	3. FEAR OF NOT KNOWING	4. DESTINATIONS
On persistence of pain, distress, or physical dysfunction, the person becomes caught in the *fear of knowing*.	The issue is avoided as long as possible. Fear of the discovery of some dread disease is further complicated by fear of the loss of dignity and personal control experienced on entering the medical system. However, as the problem continues, these fears are eventually overcome by the actual loss of control or threat of loss of control caused by the problem itself. This results in the greater *fear of not knowing* what is going on.	Seeking medical advice leads to options: Early diagnosis & effective treatment or Protracted period of unsuccessful diagnostic tests which eventually produce: a. definition of the problem and effective course of treatment or b. no satisfactory answer Diagnosis of an incurable or intractable disease, for which there is: a. a usual series of protracted treatments and drugs to modify pain and symptoms. b. no currently accepted mode of treatment	Reasonable and timely resolution or a. some life disruption and expense, but eventual relief and resolution. b. long-term dependency on medical system. Continuing tests and efforts to overcome effects of problem. or *Helplessness & Despair* a. a long-term dependency on the medical system. b. admonition to go home and live with degenerating existence.

failure to find some workable course of treatment, many patients find themselves on the pathway to helplessness based on the assumption that they are powerless to act on their own. This eventually leads to an actual breakdown of their psychological capacity to manage their lives.

THE BIOLOGY OF DESPAIR

The feelings of powerlessness and helplessness brought about by interaction with the adherents of current medical viewpoints regarding chronic disease may in themselves bring on physiological changes in the brain that further diminish the patient's ability to deal with the problem. In Lionel Tiger's new book, *Optimism: The Biology of Hope*, he points out that our outlook on the future has significant *biological* effect on the brain's production of chemicals that stimulate moods of either optimism or depression. Tiger notes:

> If we understand that social circumstances can affect the ideas people have about themselves and the world, and if in turn these ideas can influence bodily states, we begin to understand the connection between social process and medical fact.
>
> The field of neurochemistry is undergoing a compulsive upheaval, and much of the new work is directly relevant to the possibility that there is a location in the brain for good feelings about the present and the future.

In other words, once patients are told that they have an incurable disease or are left in a situation of complete dependency on the medical system, an attitude of "no future" can develop in the mind. This attitude can affect the production of chemicals called endorphins, which regulate moods and feelings of optimism or despair. Once the mood of despair becomes established, the brain endeavors to dampen the pain of the dreadful experience, producing more endorphins to "depress" the situation. The patient becomes increasingly depressed. Only a complete change of attitude about potential for the future can reverse this trend.

A NEW PATHWAY TO
ACTION AND SUCCESS

The barriers to success in finding the pathway to action are the focus on disease and the assumption that medical science must learn to identify and control each specific cause of disease. This places responsibility for action and control in the hands of professionals and leaves patients powerless to act.

As we have mentioned throughout the book, the Kaslow Program is focused not on disease but on the health and well-being of each person. We have complete confidence in the wisdom of nature and the human body. If we can learn to remove from the life choices of an individual those actions that distort the body's well-being, then nature itself will cure the disease, and we may not even know *what it was or how to treat it.*

This shift of focus and the identification of the factors that distort self-healing within the body place the option to decide on a course of action completely with the patient, creating optimism for the future, and opening up immediate steps that can change the condition.

Each patient who visits the Kaslow Centers comes to realize that:

- My illness is a result of long-term imbalances in my body resulting from nutritional habits, unresolved stress, and personal attitudes about health, and my capacity to get well. My body *is well* and *has been made ill* because I was not aware of these factors.

- My own attitudes and actions are the determinants of my future health. Medicine cannot fix me because I do not need to be fixed. I can learn to build my own health, life possibilities, and success.

- Physicians and other health care providers are valuable resources for information that can lead me to wiser choices, but I must make choices that work effectively for me.

- I can learn how my body functions, how it responds to various habits and activities, and what affects my health and well-being.

With this view in mind, it is unlikely that anyone will proceed to feelings of helplessness because each individual is in charge of the process of becoming healthy once more. It should be pointed out here that one of the wise choices a person can make is to seek traditional medical care for certain problems. However, this action can be approached in the context of self-knowledge and self-understanding rather than professional dependency. It is possible to go to a physician to seek information to solve a problem rather than to get a problem "fixed."

These new attitudes and responses are emerging because people have found old feelings and actions unproductive when dealing with chronic and degenerative diseases. As we have stated earlier, chronic disease is not an enemy to be identified and killed.

In this approach, the onset of pain, distress, and dysfunction calls for an evaluation of those life events that seem to be directly related to the episodes. Eating habits, stressful situations, unexpected life events, and lack of adequate exercise can almost always be related to the situation. Rather than fearing to know what is happening in the body, the person seeks actual working knowledge of body processes, coming to understand and be sensitive to signals from the body. Fear of not knowing dissolves as the person becomes more familiar with responses to each situation, the appropriate actions that can be taken to reverse the symptoms, and the feelings of success which such actions produce.

Patients at the Kaslow Centers are discovering that their bodies have the ability to heal years of stress and degeneration, if given the opportunity and time to do so. There is no need to "give up" and live with the problems many are facing today. We do not claim that the Kaslow Program is a panacea. But through greater self-knowledge and self-direction, identifying rejected foods, establishing a nutritional balance, relieving unresolved stress, and moving the body into new levels of flexibility and action, many are finding increased vitality, improved body flexibility, increasing control over their own lives and futures, and greater enjoyment of life. Many achieve complete wellness and return to an enjoyable life vigor.

In the next two chapters on the Kaslow Program and the workbook for health, we offer the specific steps in a plan for anyone who wants to take the pathway to health.

PART II

The
Kaslow Program

7

THE KASLOW
MEDICAL
SELF-CARE PROGRAM

THE PRECEDING CHAPTERS HAVE PROVIDED AN EXPLA-
nation of the basic concepts on which the Kaslow Program has
been built. Now, we provide you with a simulated journey
through the Center in Santa Barbara, California, introducing you
to the staff and explaining the contributions each makes. We do
this to give you a sense of the environment of support the Center
offers to many who arrive feeling that they have no power to
affect their own future.

The personal workbook for health in Chapter 8 will offer
you the opportunity to explore many of the same self-learning
and health planning activities undertaken by those who come to
Santa Barbara. You can achieve significant changes and progress
by taking the new directions suggested by this chapter and the
workbook. You will find the exercises simple in theory and easy
to attempt.

Perhaps the only barrier will be your own beliefs about your
ability to change. Your daily habits have been trained by these
beliefs. One of the primary functions of the staff in Santa Barbara
is to support the notion that each of us can change these habits
by choosing new action and that these changes can redirect our
lives toward health and well-being.

Therefore, one of our goals for this chapter is to provide you
with a sense of having been part of the family of people who

have come to Santa Barbara and found a new direction for health in their lives. As you begin your own health activity program, think of these people sharing their experiences with you. Their success can support yours.

People arriving at the Kaslow Medical Self-Care Center in Santa Barbara bring with them a wide variety of problems, symptoms, frustrations, and dysfunctions. Perhaps one out of four enters in a wheelchair or with a walker. They may have been diagnosed as having multiple sclerosis or arthritis. Others whose distress is not so outwardly obvious may arrive feeling burdened with diabetes, heart disorders, weight control problems, depression, tobacco or alcohol addictions, or any number of other conditions from which they have found no relief.

Their first impression is that of a medical setting similar to ones seen before. The Kaslow office, catty-corner to the Cottage Hospital, is surrounded by other professional offices and medical services. As one enters, the office interior also seems fairly typical of a medical office, with a reception desk and a spacious waiting room.

Soon the differences become apparent. There is no wall, either in the physical construction of the office or in the attitude of the staff, between the waiting room, the reception area, and the staff offices and examining rooms. There is no little window through which one must peer into an unseen inner sanctum where unknown and little-understood tasks are performed. A sense of openness prevails as staff people come and go through the waiting room, frequently stopping for a brief visit with a patient or family member.

This sense of openness is a symbol of the principal difference between the experience of patients here and those they have known elsewhere in the customary medical setting. The emphasis here is on patient involvement, education, and experience.

LEARNING TO SUPPORT
NATURAL SELF-REGULATION

The basic intention of the Kaslow Program is education. As we have said many times throughout the book, the program starts from the premise that chronic and degenerative dysfunctions are the result of distortions of the natural self-healing and self-regulation systems of the body. Rather than treating the symptoms of disease, the program makes the patient more aware of those factors that distort self-healing, offers insights and skills the patient and family can use at home to detect and act on difficulties before they become critical, and changes habits in nutrition, body flexibility and movement capacity, attitudes, and response to stress situations to reduce or eliminate distortions of self-regulation.

There is no Kaslow diet for arthritis, no exercise program for heart disorders, no treatment for diabetes, and so on. There are instead individualized programs to build health, which include diet, exercise, attitude changes, and relaxation techniques. The patient learns to support the self-regulation wisdom of the body. The body will then, based on its own self-regulation, alleviate or reverse the disease without direct treatment of the disease itself.

Patients discover that the steps they will take, the questions they will be asked, and the new health program they will design seem quite similar to those of their fellow patients even though the problems presented may be quite different. Each person will create a unique diet program, each will design his or her own movement and exercise program, each will have unique life situations and stress factors to explore, but this diversity has a common framework based on factors everyone must consider in order to build good health and continuing well-being.

These factors, as we have enumerated before, are metabolic rejectivity (food intolerances), general nutritional balance, relief of physical and emotional stress, effective utilization of oxygen through improved body movement and flexibility, and development of positive, self-directing attitudes about health and the future.

Each of these factors raises a series of questions, and the various aspects of the Kaslow Program are designed to answer these questions. The following lists the factors, the questions each addresses, and the aspects of the program directed to those questions. Look these over and then we will take you on an imaginary visit to the Kaslow Center, where you'll gain an experience shared by so many others.

Metabolic rejectivity.   Do I habitually eat foods my body cannot tolerate? Am I aware of my body's response to these foods? Can I learn to identify these responses and plan a diet that does not include foods harmful to my health?

The aspects of the program explaining how to find the answers to these questions are the Diet Survey, the Nonprocessed Carbohydrate Tolerance Test, the Resting Fast, and the Response Diet testing diary.

General nutritional balance.   Do my food choices represent variety or lack of variety? Are there a small number of foods I eat consistently, limiting my choices? Is my diet skewed in some unbalanced direction? Do I eat fresh foods or mostly processed and refined foods? How much sugar is in my regular diet? Do my food choices provide a basic supply of the nutrients needed for action energy, body building and maintenance, and successful self-regulation?

The diet survey, nutritional counseling, diet planning after the food rejectivity testing, and stool analysis are all aspects of the program designed to provide answers to these questions.

Relief of physical and emotional stress.   What situations in my life may be burdening me with unresolved stress? Can I gain some skills for recognizing and relaxing these stresses? Are there particularly sensitive areas of my body where stress energy is being retained? Can this stress energy be released and redirected?

The Stress/Stamina Balancing Program, Response Point Therapy, and the Dialogue in Human Concerns deal with some aspect of the resolution of stress to rebalance the body.

Body movement, flexibility, and effective oxygen use.   Can my body be more capable of movement and flexibility? Can I exercise regularly in a way that stimulates my cardiovascular system and promotes greater vitality? What does my breathing and my body's capacity to convert oxygen signify for my health? Can I be free to walk and care for myself again (if I am now disabled)?

The Stress/Stamina Balancing Program addresses these questions and offers individualized answers to give each person new directions in working toward movement and flexibility.

Positive, self-directing attitudes. How do my life choices affect the course of my disease? Are the decisions and actions necessary for improvement in my hands or am I dependent on medical professionals? What sense do I have of my body? Is my body a failure I fear and hate because it is inhabited by an enemy, my disease? What will make it possible for me to get well? Am I willing to get well?

All aspects of the Kaslow Program and all members of the staff deal with these questions in every meeting with patients and families. Though the questions may not always be asked specifically, they are behind every activity a patient undertakes at the Center. The staff's assumption that everyone can and will improve as a result of new life choices based on greater self-awareness is a fundamental part of an environment in which the whole program operates. More specifically, the Dialogue in Human Concerns deals with these questions in a direct, open way.

Of the several aspects of the Kaslow Program just mentioned, the following options will be available to you in the workbook that follows in Chapter 8, either exactly as they are presented at the Center, or in a form slightly modified to make them self-explanatory for ready use:

- Metabolic Rejectivity—diet survey, resting fast, response diet testing diary

- General Nutritional Balance—diet survey, diet planning

- Stress—some aspects of the Stress/Stamina Balancing Program and the Dialogue in Human Concerns are offered in several of the workbook exercises

- Body Movement and Flexibility—several exercises are included for getting in touch with and improving your capacity for movement and oxygen use. These have been drawn from the Stress/Stamina Balancing Program

- Attitudes—our entire book supports the development of positive self-directing attitudes about your future well-being. The workbook includes an attitude survey, the self-awareness survey, and other exercises designed to give you support as you change your daily health routine.

Simply because of the nature of the required interaction with staff, we have no way to offer the following other aspects of the program in a workbook: the nonprocessed carbohydrate tolerance test, stool and hair analysis, response point therapy, and the direct counseling sessions on nutrition, sharing in human concerns, and stress/stamina balancing. They are described in this chapter so that you can see how they fit into the Kaslow Program.

As much as we could, we have endeavored to communicate the essence of the activities to you in the workbook and in this chapter. We are assured that the activities you can undertake on your own after reading this book offer every opportunity for significant change in your health and your future.

A WALK THROUGH THE KASLOW PROGRAM

Orientation

We have spoken of the anxiety, fear, and mistrust all too frequently associated with medical care today. Recognizing this, the Kaslow Center begins each week with a general orientation session.

In this one-and-a-half hour meeting, newcomers have an opportunity to become familiar with the Center, meet some of the practitioners with whom they will be working, and relieve initial anxieties usually present when someone moves into new circumstances.

Staff members briefly describe each phase of the Program and encourage questions and open discussion. Not only do the patients have this opportunity to know the staff, but the staff also has a brief introduction to each new patient and develops a sense for personal needs that will be useful in later interaction.

Metabolic Rejectivity

In Chapter 3, we described the clinical experience on which this hypothesis is based. The combination of the body's inability to metabolize effectively carbohydrates and the habitual eating of foods rejected by the body sets up a continuing spiral of stress (the hypoglycemic response) and harassment of sites of damaged tissue (the immune system's lymphocyte response).

There are four steps in the Kaslow Program's efforts to teach patients how best to manage their food choices to avoid the consequences of metabolic rejectivity, that is what we have labeled chronic disease. These steps are the Diet Survey, the Nonprocessed Carbohydrate Tolerance Test, the Resting Fast, and the Response Diet Testing diary. The Diet Survey will be explored in the following section, which deals with general nutritional balance.

The Nonprocessed Carbohydrate Tolerance Test

This test, which takes the better part of a day (see Figure 3.1 showing the 6½ hour responses), is more than a laboratory test to gain information from within the body. It is also an experience offering each patient insights into physical, psychological, and emotional responses to food.

The medical reason for the test is to determine each patient's blood sugar and immune system response to a significant intake of fructose, the natural sugar found in fruit. The individual reason for the test is so each patient may have a direct experience of the body's responses to food.

Each patient is asked not to eat or drink anything between dinner and morning arrival at the Center. Prior to the beginning of the test, a "base line" or fasting blood sample is taken to establish the blood sugar level and lymphocyte count. The patient then slowly eats 3 oranges, 6 dates, and 1 banana—about 100 grams of natural fructose. Two parallel activities follow. The patient keeps a running diary of feelings, moods, sensations, and psychological responses, and a series of six additional blood samples are drawn at one-hour intervals starting one and one-half hours after eating.

Although the blood samples provide valuable clinical information about the individual's metabolic responses to this meal, by far the most important lesson is learned from the actual monitoring of body and mind responses. For the first time, many people realize that what they eat and drink has a direct and immediate affect on how they feel, both physically and psychologically. Responses during the six- to seven-hour test period range from high to low, ecstatic to depressed.

As we mentioned before, the most significant realization of many patients is an experience of an acute, intense episode of the symptoms of the chronic ailment from which they seek relief. This establishes at a very personal level the direct link between food habits and the problem and illustrates that learning different choices more acceptable to the body can reverse the disease process.

Patients going through the nonprocessed carbohydrate tolerance test are frequently amazed as they learn to sense their own bodies and "read" responses and feelings resulting from the test.

I'm feeling that dull ache that comes and goes in my shoulder.

I feel lousy, I'd like to lie down and take a nap.

I'm lightheaded and dizzy and feel nervous and excited [early in the test during rapid rise in blood sugar].

I feel listless and tired [later, when blood sugar falls].

My hands are stiff and I'm having trouble doing the writing in my diary.

Each patient gains a new sense of awareness of responses to foods and possibilities for new food combinations to create positive feelings and responses.

The Resting Fast

After the six and one-half hour carbohydrate tolerance test, the metabolism of the body is usually in an unbalanced state induced by the intake of more than 100 grams of fructose and the subsequent physical and mental responses. To properly prepare for individual food testing for rejected foods, there must be time for the body to regain balance. One of the most effective ways to regain metabolic balance in the body is to *do nothing* for a short period. The internal self-regulation systems are then free to reestablish normal function without any interruption from food requiring processing. Therefore, each patient embarks on a 48-hour distilled water fast.

Distilled water is recommended because tap water is usually loaded with chemicals or may contain excess minerals in some areas. Even though tap water might not aggravate the body when taken with foods in the normal routine, the body almost always considers it unsuitable when it is the only substance being ingested. Unless you know that the water in your area is chemically free and fairly balanced with natural minerals, we recommend distilled water for all consumption (including cooking).

Many people, especially those suffering chronic illness, may be afraid to fast. They feel that not eating may weaken their already failing body. Surprisingly, the reverse may be true. The foods they are eating may be perpetuating the symptoms and the problem. Not eating may ameliorate symptoms.

In our experience, seven out of ten patients feel some relief from their symptoms as a result of the fast alone. After the experience of the body's response to the carbohydrate tolerance test, this added awareness of the body's capacity to relax and rebound when it is left alone for a short fasting period serves to illustrate further to many the direct relationship between food habits and their illness or dysfunction. The fasting experience proves of such value to some patients that they decide to set aside one or two days each week for distilled water fasts. This allows the body to rest and reset its self-regulation systems on a regular basis.

During the fasting period, we advise those experiencing any disabling illness not to undertake strenuous physical activity. It is essential to allow the body to rest and regain its balance and to reach a state of relaxation.

We do not propose extended fasts or juice and limited food fasts. After the body has a brief opportunity to rest, it is best to keep it active as well as nourished and flowing. The self-regulation systems will then handle any imbalances that may arise through the use of their natural processes.

Response Diet Testing

One of the cornerstones of the Kaslow Program is the Metabolic Rejectivity Syndrome concept which says that chronically ill people are especially sensitive to certain foods but continue to eat these foods, unaware of their body's reaction to them. The body's response to these nontolerated and aggravating foods triggers the immune system's scavenger cells (lymphocytes), which move into the bloodstream and then into the body tissues to remove the unwanted substances. Consistently eating these unwanted foods eventually fatigues the immune response; it becomes erratic and harasses stressed tissues in the body. The sites of these stressed tissues then become the symptoms noticed by the patient with chronic disease.

In order to reverse this degenerating process, it is necessary to identify each food an individual's body cannot tolerate and eliminate that food from the diet. As we mentioned earlier, these foods so identified may have been considered as nutritious, for example, oranges or broccoli, and thus were eaten conscientiously as part of a good "basic four" diet.

Metabolic Rejectivity sets the Kaslow Program apart from all formula diet plans for chronic disease that are based on limited, prescribed diets to fight the disease. The attempt to manage the function of the body by formula strategies is unwise in our view because these diets usually limit and encourage the patient to eat a very few foods chosen to *fix* the current situation, not to achieve long-term balance. In addition, the diet may contain foods that are the *cause of the problem* for that individual.

Another factor is that because of the limited food choices, a person may actually develop a rejectivity response to some "good" food eaten repeatedly within the framework of the diet. Our experience is that such diets may work for about three to five weeks, then diminish in value or become *harmful*. The desired outcome of the high-variety diet worked out by each patient in the Kaslow Program is *rebalance* of the body, not *correction* of the disease. If the body is balanced and nourished by a diet containing a variety of nutrients but not containing rejected foods, the body will then correct the disease on its own.

The process of testing foods is a simple concept. First, foods that are known through our experience to have a high risk of rejectivity are not tested during the early test period. These high risk foods are all foods containing refined sugar, processed dairy products (cheeses, yogurt, homogenized milk), the gluten grains (wheat, barley, rye, oats), fruits (citrus and other tree-grown fruits), and chocolate. The dairy products, grains, and fruits may be tested later in the process. Refined sugar, refined flour, processed foods, and chocolate are permanently eliminated from the diet.

Without these high-risk foods, the foods that are tested are more likely to be safe, allowing the body to recover its healing capabilities without stress. Each person works from an intensive list of foods including fresh vegetables, chicken, meat, and fish proteins, roots and tubers, nuts and seeds, sprouts, and so on. A complete list and description of this process is given in Chapter 8 in the section on "Response Food Testing."

Twelve foods are selected for the first three days of the test. Only one food is eaten per meal, four meals per day, using only pure, creamery sweet butter and sea salt as condiments (no sauces, spices, ketchup, salad dressings, etc.). During the fourth and fifth day, meals are made up of combinations of 8 small portions of these 12 foods, omitting any food to which the person has had a negative response. Testing 4 more *new* foods per day for the next 3 days will provide another 12 foods to combine for the next 8-food-test meal. This procedure is carried on for a number of sessions.

During the food testing period, the individual keeps a Response Diet Diary, recording physical, emotional, and psychological responses to each food. The signals may vary and a food may need to be retested if there is a stress situation that may take place unexpectedly, such as receiving an unpleasant phone call thirty minutes after eating. Usually, though, the signals are clear and distinct. If the body does not like the food, feedback is strong and obvious: headaches, depression or anxiety, pain, fatigue, drowsiness and possible full-blown recurrence of chronic symptoms. Reactions to foods will occur at differing times after eating but, we have found, are almost always apparent to the individual within two to three hours if there is a modest development of self-awareness.

The process of testing usually takes from two to four weeks as the person savors the variety of foods and picks the winners. The final result of the testing is a *personal* list of foods the body enjoys, a *list of foods the body rejects*, and a far keener sense of how the body works. Paying personal attention to your body for a month returns great dividends and is bound to change your perception of yourself.

From the list of desirable foods, the individual can now prepare menus to include a *wide variety* of foods chosen with discretion to assure the body's supply of personally essential nutrients. (See Chapter 5 and its lists of foods providing each essential nutrient.)

Patients are de-addicted to smoking during the total program and the food testing. Smoking provides no value to the body whatsoever and serves no function other than to distort homeostatic self-regulation systems. Smoking is related to many chronic illnesses, not just the heart and lung disorders with which it has been popularly identified. One of the principal benefits many patients enjoy from the balancing process of the nutritional and Response Point Therapy programs is a *loss of the craving for cigarettes.* These cravings and addictions are but symptoms of imbalance in the body. Smoking de-addiction occurs *without withdrawal symptoms* on this total program.

A Note from Chelsea Reimers, Nutrition Counselor

A significant factor in success with the food testing program is the available support. Out-of-towners who are surrounded by activities here at the Center in Santa Barbara do very well while they are here but seem to have some difficulty keeping up with the program when they return home. Then there are the local patients, who are continuing their usual life routine while food testing. The patients have a harder time getting started, have a slower response to the program in terms of improvement, but usually reach a par with the others in the long run. If readers can arrange to do the food testing with one or two others who want to share the process, it will probably be easier to stay on the program.

Our observation of these two types of patients makes it clear that there are two major requirements for success in nutritional rebalancing: being able to change long-standing habits and having people around you who are willing to support these changes and sometimes put up with unusual food preparation routines. Since long-term habits have contributed so much to the problem in the first place, people need to recognize these concerns and be prepared to work with them. It's not just a matter of foods, it's also a matter of willingness, persistence, and attitude. *This program has worked successfully for everyone we know who has been willing to stick with it.* Our "failures" are people who cannot make the adjustments in their lives and habits. It's their choice to make.

R.L.G., a man of about 60, came in with a diagnosis of multiple sclerosis. His physical problems were repeated falling due to poor balance, right foot drop and numbness. His total weakness bothered him mostly. He had been eating the standard American diet: a variety of meats, milk and eggs, several cups of coffee daily, citrus fruits four to six times a week, large amounts of white bread and jelly, and he also frequented Mexican restaurants. His attitude was, "I have MS and that's that!"

His stool analysis showed incomplete digestion of vegetables. His food testing indicated rejection of steak and corn, a staple of Mexican foods. He didn't want to give up steak, and he wavered on and off his program.

Eventually, he began to recognize the benefits of the program and integrated it into his lifestyle. Working with Gordon Hendrickson (the stress/stamina consultant at the Center), R.L.G. took up swimming and began to be more active. With his wife's support, he stayed on his new diet, gave up corn and beef, and rebalanced his food intake without sugars and coffee. He is now walking and swimming and has become positive, even enthusiastic in his approach. He's now on the pathway to restoring his health. He no longer thinks of himself as an MS patient!

Victoria, aged 55, a diagnosed diabetic for 10 years, had also been diagnosed as having multiple sclerosis about a month before she came to the Center. She is an interesting example of prescribed diets and later problems. Ten years ago, when she learned about her diabetes, doctors had told her to refrain primarily from sugar consumption. Her food habits became based on easy-to-prepare convenience foods that seemed to fit into the doctor's recommendations. Her diet was the usual high-protein type, was beef at least once a day, and plenty of eggs, margarine, and dairy products. She ate few vegetables, only avoiding onions, spices, cabbage, and beans because they created gas. She ate fruits, nuts, dairy products, and, occasionally, chocolate but almost no grains or cereals. On her diet survey this added up to a distorted intake of foods supplying basic vitamins and minerals and a diet rich in fat and simple carbohydrates but lacking in complex carbohydrates.

The basic program of Response Diet Testing eliminated fruits, dairy products, and chocolate from her diet. She discovered a nontolerance of potatoes, beets, and corn, especially when these foods were eaten in combination with each other. Rebalancing of her vitamin and mineral intake smoothed out the gas problems she had been experiencing and ameliorated those symptoms. Within a few weeks, her demeanor began to change, she felt more cheerful and in control of her life, and she was on the road to enjoying an active life again.

Typical of a far different problem was a young woman of 29 who came to us chronically depressed and emotionally shaken. Food had become an obsession with her. She ate six meals a day and literally designed each meal according to a master formula. She was seeking a "food prescription" that would solve all her life problems. She made a research project out of eating and was becoming a near specialist in biochemistry. She was woefully confused and overwhelmed by all the information and misinformation in books and shop talk about nutrition and health. She was a high-speed rambling talker and almost bowled us over with her machine-gun questions and comments about foods, supplements, vitamins, and the like. Her problem was not entirely one of nutrition. She spent some time with Juliet (our Dialogue in Human Concerns counselor) so that she could get a clearer understanding of her emotional anxieties about foods.

Just as we seek balance in foods, exercise, and stress, we must seek balance in our approach to these issues. Food was not at the root of this woman's problem. Her obsessive interest in foods was a symptom of deeper uncertainties and confusion about how she might make her life successful. What we are saying is that food response testing is not some magic process that will solve every problem known to humanity. It must be kept in perspective. We want to listen to and care for our patients as much as we work to help them rebalance their personal nutritional deficiencies and excesses.

A Note from Dr. Kaslow about
Vitamin and Mineral Supplementation

Some people may wonder about "megavitamin" therapies and how we approach that issue. As a result of the testing at the Center, we do discover some individuals in serious deficiency states for certain essential substances. In perhaps the only prescriptive part of our program, we prescribe large doses of some vitamins for these individuals to restore body balance.

We must add that these doses are tested in the same way that individual foods are tested. They are tried, one substance at a time, so that the individual can assess the body's response as in the food testing. We cannot predict with any certainty how any individual will respond to a megadosage of vitamins and we need this direct feedback before continuing the process. We have found that about 10 percent of our patients reject certain vitamin supplements.

For persons developing their own nutrition programs, we cannot recommend dashing off to a health food store, stocking up on large quantities of vitamins and minerals, and spending a lot of money on food supplements. Each person should develop a personal plan, based on the rules of food tolerance/nontolerance, wide variety, freshness, and preparation we discussed in Chapter 5.

Should you decide to use any supplemental vitamins or minerals based on some body signal (see the deficiency symptoms listed for each vitamin and mineral in Table 5.2) keep written track of the signal in your Response Diary. If it diminishes or goes away, you may be able to reduce your intake of the supplement or stop altogether. Respond to present circumstances, not to your past image of the problem.

General Nutritional Balance

In Chapter 5, we provided basic suggestions for achieving a balanced diet. Good food is natural, not refined or processed, does not include refined sugar, is eaten as fresh as possible, is prepared in modest quantity per meal, is never overcooked, includes a variety of foods from the several food categories, is enjoyed in an appropriate setting, and does not include foods your body is rejecting.

Tables 5.2 and 5.3, listing the components of various foods, provide a planning base for choosing foods that will include all the needed nutritional elements. But before you plan what you should eat, it is helpful to take stock of what you're eating now. The Diet Survey aids in this process.

The Diet Survey

Each person who arrives at the Center completes a Diet Survey. The survey is reproduced in Chapter 8 and you can complete one yourself. The purpose of this survey is twofold: (1) to provide a discussion base for an extended interview with the nutrition counselor, and (2) to serve as a mirror to reflect back to the individual sometimes surprising information about personal food habits.

We all know what we eat, but we rarely stop to look at the overall picture of the food choices we make, the frequency of each choice, the types of foods we may choose as favorites, or those we may leave out altogether. Participating in the survey provides a self-analysis revealing a great deal about food habits and choices.

Persons who have not previously explored planned nutrition are usually surprised by what they learn from this simple survey.

There are many foods listed on here that I never eat.

It looks like I eat the same thing all the time.

I wasn't aware that I drink so much orange juice [coffee, milk].

Yes, I eat essentially the same breakfast each morning.

I guess I snack more than I should.

I certainly eat more sugar and sugared foods than I realized.

During interviews, we discover that many patients do not list between-meal snacks on the survey: "I thought you were just surveying meals, I didn't know this other stuff (chips, candy, soft drinks, pastries) was food." They may be right, in a sense, but the body must process everything taken in.

Nutrition Counseling

This interview, early in the Program, offers an opportunity for the patient to see, perhaps for the first time, the overall picture of his or her diet habits. When you complete your diet survey, you can ask yourself the same questions that we ask in our interviews. Are there a variety of foods eaten, or is the diet limited? Is there a balance among the several food groups, or are most foods in just a few categories? What kind of meals are eaten —regular, stable meals or quick snacks and fast-food meals? Are some of the same foods eaten every day or more than once a day? A review of these questions, easily revealed by the Diet Survey questionnaire and drawn out during the counseling interview, offers insights into attitudes about foods, how foods are chosen and prepared, and the physical, mental, and emotional role foods play in the daily activity of the individual.

The counselor can then assess the individual's awareness of the relationship of food habits to current or potential problems. Many of the patients coming to the Center have not considered their food habits to be directly involved in their illness or general dysfunction. It takes some time and thought to begin to make the connection between what you eat and the condition of the mind and body. The counselor gains a background foundation during this interview for a teaching relationship with each person.

During the interview, the counselor begins the educational process based on each person's understanding of his or her nutritional situation. The end goal is to achieve two objectives:

1. To identify and remove from the individual's diet those foods the body cannot tolerate which are triggering overstimulated immune responses (metabolic rejectivity).

2. To have each individual create a productive diet, based on the suggestions made earlier in this section and in Chapter 5, that supports the body's needs for action energy, body building and maintenance, and the process of self-regulation.

A Note from Chelsea Reimers

In my discussion with patients, I am interested in three aspects of nutrition: content, habit, and style. My experience has been that almost all nutrition discussions focus on content alone. Of course, what we eat is very important to our wellbeing, but we must also consider the frequency of eating each food, size of meals, snacking, how many meals are eaten each day, heavy foods or light foods, attitudes while eating (rushed and anxious or calm and enjoyable), and the general importance of foods in the person's lifestyle. During interviews, I gain a sense of how each person thinks about foods and the role these foods play in many life habits.

Content. Relative to content, we want to assure that the individual can learn to create a diet providing all the essential nutrients. Since there are so many possible choices of foods, and personal likes and dislikes are important, we offer lists of foods by type which people can choose from (see Chapter 8). Then, our focus is more on what might be left off their diet plan, since within the lists the choices are up to the individual.

Our general rules for content are (1) no refined sugar, (2) very little or no processed foods containing additives and colorings, (3) variety—choosing many different foods and not repeating foods more frequently than every four or five days, (4) foods as fresh as possible, and (5) reading of all labels to be aware of the contents of foods you buy.

Persons who arrive following some fixed diet supposedly designed to treat the disease start from scratch just like anyone else, learning as they go to support what their body likes and wants rather than trying to fix their problem through nutrition.

Of course, in the Response Diet Testing, each person discovers those specific foods that the body cannot tolerate and are causing pain and dysfunction. I should mention that many of these foods are not "bad" or processed foods. They include almost all foods, but the rejectivity is unique to each individual. There seems to be no predictable formula and each person must learn which foods are personally rejected by the body.

Habit. A person's eating habits can give immediate clues to the role food plays in his life. Someone who snacks on candy or chips, likes lots of sugar and salt, usually has to keep going all the time. This type of person is usually "speedy" and nervous and may be using these foods to fill an emotional need.

People who are always busy and eat on the run, never stopping to enjoy a relaxed meal with an appropriate appreciation for the food and sustenance, will probably be suffering from problems with digestion and assimilation. They also have a tendency to eat foods that are quick and easy to prepare, fast-foods and the so-called junk foods. This shows how advertising, peer values, and social custom influence our eating habits. There is no easier convenience food than raw vegetables. It's fairly easy to have a snack of celery sticks, carrot slices, cocktail tomatoes, broccoli or cauliflower for munching on the job or for a light lunch. Inexpensive and requiring no preparation, these foods are fresh and unprocessed. Yet, few people would think of such a snack for fear others might joke or look askance at them. As people become more nutritionally aware, they begin to see the ease and value of these easy-to-carry foods.

Habit also includes the variety, or lack of variety, each person chooses. Our diet surveys show that many people eat only a very limited number of foods day after day. Many times people will eat the same breakfast and lunch five days a week, then shift to a similar repetition of other foods on the weekend. I have spoken to some people who have eaten the same breakfast every day for more than 15 or 20 years. If these limited choices contain some foods rejected by the body, this repetitive eating pattern can cause serious problems. The body may even learn to reject foods eaten that frequently, even though not originally sensitive to them.

Style. Style of eating has changed for many in recent years. Not too many years ago, a Norman Rockwell painting evoked thoughts of the American family saying grace over an abundant Sunday meal. As corny as this may seem, this sense of security and serenity associated with a meal can be important to how the body responds to foods. Easier digestion and more effective assimilation will occur in a relaxed, at ease body. Our bodies cannot be separated from our attitudes and emotions!

How we feel about the people we are eating with, how we feel about our work, ourselves, and how we regard the food before us will all have some effect on the body's interaction with the food. If we relax before meals, take a moment to consider the many people and an abundant nature that placed the food before us, and be thankful for the food and our lives, our enjoyment and actual use of the food will be enhanced. Families should consider whether mealtimes become times of argument or

distress and how much everyone enjoys or avoids coming together for a meal. All these factors are important in our relationship to food.

Another comment on food style concerns those who make a
personal research crusade out of nutrition. They become obsessed with all the new schemes and ideas, must analyze the
details of very food, and plan their daily menu as if it were the
chemical formula for a manufacturing plant. This limitation of
food experiences to content formulation costs these people the
enjoyment of preparing, savoring, and exploring meals in most
cases. The pleasant sensations of handling foods, savoring the
cooking odors, and sharing their richness and flavor with others
during a warm, pleasant meal is lost to concern about percentages
and quotas. I think that's too bad. Content is important, but food
is nourishment in more ways than content. One of the outcomes
of this obsession can be separation and isolation from others
who can't understand a "food nut." I think it's unfortunate if
food habits are built on isolation and loneliness.

This brings up another point. People who are exploring new
food habits are going to experience change in their lives. This
process of change is difficult to do on your own. It's more fun
and easier to keep on the track if you are sharing your journey
with others. I would recommend to people that they find a
friend or two with whom to share the Diet Survey, Response
Diet planning, and perhaps even to compare their Response Diet
Testing diary from time to time.

Stool Analysis

If you are working on this Program on your own or with
your own physician and your difficulties include intestinal dysfunction, accumulating fatigue, or persistent degeneration of your
body (continuing weight loss and loss of mobility and function)
in the face of a reasonable and nutritious diet, a comprehensive
stool analysis may offer worthwhile information. A good stool
survey will indicate your body's capacity to absorb nutrients
from your food. A stool analysis is not essential to the effective
use of the Program, but it may prove useful if attempts to change
the course of your difficulty do not seem to be producing results.

The stool analysis may show that some digestive enzyme imbalance exists in the intestinal tract that needs special attention.

An analysis of stool content can explain a great deal about the digestive process. It is possible to eat a reasonably balanced and nutritious diet and yet receive inadequate nutrition from good food because the *functional* ability of the digestive system has been distorted by food rejectivity, stress, lack of oxygen, or general fatigue. Much more common, failure of the digestive process is attributable to deficiencies of vitamins and digestive enzymes resulting from unbalanced food choices. Add to this the problems of stress, food rejectivity, and general body fatigue, and the stage is set for a long-term process that ultimately results in some form of degenerative disease.

At the Kaslow Center, a comprehensive stool analysis is used as a check on the efficiency of the digestive process, the nature and content of the bacterial flora in the bowels, and the presence of infection or inflammation of the intestine in each patient. In a few extreme cases, patients whose digestive system may not be supportive to the nutritional needs of the body as a whole may have to take digestive enzyme supplements or other supportive supplementation.

In the workbook chapter (Chapter 8), we have included a special commentary on constipation, a common problem easily solved through nutrition and exercise.

Stress/Movement, Flexibility, and Oxygen Use/Attitudes

Earlier, in the initial outline of this chapter, we spoke of those aspects of the program involving unresolved physical and emotional stress; body movement, flexibility, effective oxygen use; and positive, self-directing attitudes.

There are three aspects of the program remaining to be explored and it is difficult to specify exactly how these aspects "fit under" the above categories. All aspects of the Kaslow Program are interrelated. In the case of Response Point Therapy, the Stress/Stamina Balancing Program, and Dialogue in Human Concerns, each staff member is looking at, and providing service in, several of the above categories *concurrently*.

Response Point Therapy

Response Point Therapy (RPT) has been developed at the Kaslow Center based on Dr. Kaslow's study of acupuncture concepts. In traditional Chinese medical thought, life energy (Chi) circulates through the body, passing through 14 pathways, or meridians, associated with specific functions. Each meridian represents an organ (heart, lung, kidney, spleen, large intestine, etc.) or a function (circulation/sex, conception vessel, etc.) and is also symbolic of the balance of complementary energies within the world—yin and yang. *Yin* is characterized as feminine, light, negative (in the electromagnetic sense, not the value sense), intuitive, and passive; *yang* as masculine, heavy, positive, intellectual, and active. In this view of life, these energies must flow in complementary interaction with one another and achieve periodic balance.

The ancient practice of acupuncture involved the insertion of very small needles at specified points on each meridian to tonify (energize) meridians perceived to be deficient in energy or to sedate meridians perceived to be overactive.

Imagine a large field to be irrigated with water through a series of channels and ditches. Picture little gates and valves at various places throughout the field to regulate water flow and assure that the whole field is soaked. As the water flows around, the farmer watches the gates and valves and makes appropriate adjustments, directing more water to dry areas and slowing the flow to soaked areas.

Think of your body as an energy system similar to the irrigated field. Then imagine that nutritional imbalance, stress, and lack of exercise have caused some of your gates and valves to malfunction, staying closed when they should open, sometimes opening when they should close. Parts of your body will become flooded while others cry for water.

The function of the acupuncture treatment is to gently push body energy through the system of gates and valves and loosen them up for more productive function. Once the gates and valves are functioning again, the system relaxes and finds itself easier to maintain.

The Chinese felt that all pain and dysfunction in the body resulted from energy flow along these meridians which was blocked, dammed up behind closed gates (to use our water anal-ogy). Once the energy was released, the pain would subside. Our clinical experience validates this, although there are a number of other processes taking place at the same time, so that it is hard to pin down a "cause-effect" relationship.

There are about 350 acupuncture points on the body along the 14 meridians. Marilyn Hanson, R.N., the Response Point Therapist (Res PT), performs what is called a total tonification, touching each of these points with a minute charge of electrical energy (rather than inserting a needle). As Marilyn watches the response of each patient, she discovers points that are more sensitive than others. These points indicate specific blockages along that meridian.

Discovering these points serves two purposes: It signals the points to be given further attention in future sessions, and it pro-vides clues to systems in the body that are malfunctioning.

Two to five follow-up sessions are usually scheduled for any patient with significantly sensitive points. Generally, after the sessions, the points are no longer sensitive. A more even energy flow, almost always accompanied by a relief of symptoms, results. Patients can obtain a small electrical stimulator to take home for use if symptoms recur.

As a direct example of the success of this therapy, persons experiencing bladder incontinence, as a result of a neurogenic system dysfunction, will almost always be responsive on points along the bladder meridian. Treatment of these response points alleviates the incontinence in nearly every case. Persons with strong food, smoking, or alcohol addictions will respond to what are called the "addiction points" on the ears. Treatment of these addiction points has been very successful in eliminating the crav-ing for the addictive substance, *without* the usual withdrawal symptoms that many patients fear so much.

A Note from Marilyn Hanson, R.N.

Each patient is different. Chelsea [the nutrition counselor] and I probably spend more time with patients than the other staff members simply because of the way the program schedule works out. We provide plenty of assurance and give a great deal of support. Most important we *listen* to their anxieties and con-cerns. Many people are in deep need of someone to listen.

A great many patients have a hard time believing they can improve, even though they come to the Center for that reason. Ralph, 52, came in with severe low back pain. He couldn't bend over to tie his shoes, couldn't lift anything, and because of the intense pain had been unable to work for about two years as a TV repairman.

In our initial discussion he couldn't believe that his back pain could be related to his heavy smoking (two or three packs a day) and his diet. There is an "addiction point" on the front edge of the upper ear. Ralph's was remarkably responsive. We convinced him of the need to shift from his diet of overprocessed foods. He was given six Response Point treatments, with special attention to his auricular addiction points. He stopped smoking as a test to see what would happen. With the six treatments, change of diet, and no-smoking plan, his back pain went away! He's working again now and keeps in touch just to tell us how good he feels.

These simple but direct techniques sometimes surprise even us. We tended to think of ourselves as working primarily with people suffering from long-term illnesses found most frequently in older people. That's not always true.

Recently, a couple came in with their 11-year-old daughter. She had been climbing in the rafters of the garage and had fallen onto the concrete floor, causing a serious brain injury. She was essentially a complete invalid when she arrived. The parents had been told ignominiously that she was nothing more than a "vegetable," curled up in a fetal position in a wheelchair, with tubes to feed her and a urinary catheter because she could not control her bladder. She had no limb movement and could not speak. Their neurologist thought he had convinced the parents she was essentially a vegetable and had suggested long-term pacifying medications. The parents were furious and would not give up. They told the attending physicians their daughter was not a pet to be put to sleep.

Reviewing this previous medical program we immediately saw that the liquid nourishment she had been receiving was grossly unbalanced. We reviewed the diet with her parents and instituted a variety of special formulas to bolster her recovery or healing systems.

Although it was difficult to communicate with her and re-assure her, we began a program of total tonification Response Point Therapy. Some points were very responsive and she would mumble when they were stimulated. I found this disturbing since I did not want her to feel that I might hurt her. However, these mumbles were the only sounds she had made for some time and we felt it imperative to continue. She told us with her eyes that we must, and she could sense that we cared and that something was happening within her body.

After three RPT sessions, each treatment carried out ever so much longer than with most patients, her body began to respond. Her legs and arms relaxed into a more normal sitting position in the wheelchair. Some arm and leg muscle use re-turned. We removed the nasal tube and the bladder catheter; she began to take nourishment by mouth and could control her bladder. When she arrived at the office for her fourth visit, she spoke her own name! We laughed and cried, and I ran about the halls telling everyone.

Barbara A., in her mid-forties, came in with typical multiple sclerosis difficulties: loss of balance, blurred vision, and numb-ness of the extremities. Since shortly after her diagnosis a year before, she had been in a wheelchair most of the time.

During the nutrition counseling and Response Diet testing, she discovered a strong adverse reaction to chicken and eggs, both foods she ate frequently. According to our plan, she elim-inated these foods from her diet while she was following the Response Point Therapy program.

During the initial two-hour process of total tonification, I have plenty of time to talk to patients and reassure them, buoy their self-confidence. I spoke with Barbara about the structure of her nervous system as we worked, likening it to a telephone system with messages buzzing about. I told her we needed to uncross the wires and get the calls through and that she could visualize this, making images in her mind of successful messages from her brain reaching the muscles in her arms and legs.

Usually, I can find about 16 points on someone's body that are especially reactive. Barbara and I worked together to identify these points, which we gave special attention, spending about 15 min-utes on these response points. She returned for five additional sessions during the next two weeks. We worked intensively on these special points and continued to encourage her imagery of the internal telephone system.

With her growing self-confidence and reaffirmation of self-control, as well as because of the diet changes, Barbara was walking within two weeks! She has been in touch since and continues to improve.

Stress/Stamina Balancing Program

This aspect of the Kaslow Program has two objectives: first, to establish for each patient a more effective understanding of what he or she *can do* with body movement, shifting focus off what cannot be done; and second to work out a reasonable program of exercise and movement to regain muscle flexibility, which always improves oxygen utilization.

Everyone needs to exercise to maintain body vitality and health. However, if someone is experiencing pain or significant functional impairment, the usual response is to stop using that portion of the body or to restrict its use. Once the use of an arm, hand, leg or any portion of the body has been restricted for a long period, it does not occur to us that part of the problem may be that we have forgotten how that part functions. Damage to the nervous system or to muscle tissues, plus the memory of earlier pain and distress, may somehow erase the memory of how to move. If we do not retrain and reorient the nerves with the muscles, they atrophy and become weak and unreliable. Anger at the failure of the body to perform expected tasks, externalization of the problem ("How did this happen to me?"), and assuming the role of a helpless victim all stand in the way of a person trying to regain control of the impaired nonworking parts of the body.

Once the rejected foods have been removed from the diet and nutritional balance regained, the body as a whole begins to feel good again. As emotional stresses are recognized and relieved, the individual wants to move on to new activities. If the body won't work, frustration can mount. Now is the time to "relearn" use of previously distressed nerves and muscles.

The process requires patience and consistency. When we learned to walk as a child, it took months. Because someone once knew how to perform routine actions, they can become upset because the body fails to respond instantly to the desire for action. Consider that the body *does not know how* anymore and training must begin again.

In addition to comfortable movement and flexibility, the body needs to be able to convert adequate oxygen for all metabolic functions. For anyone concerned with maintaining good health, an efficient heart/lung/circulatory system is essential. People with long-term functional impairment and chronic ailments have an added need to increase their vital limits and regain good health. Breathing more deeply, moving the body in regular rhythmic and steady exercise that stimulates the heart/lung/circulation system, is one of the most direct routes to improved vitality and feeling better. The wave of interest in jogging and aerobics is probably the most important factor in the decrease of heart disorders and strokes of the last ten years.

Everyone can move and breathe to some extent, even if there is still some dysfunction to be worked out. A regular regime of breathing and exercise is a boon to the body. In the Chapter 8 we have included a number of suggestions for persons of different ranges of physical ability.

A Note from Gordon Hendrickson, Stress/Stamina Balancing Consultant

I started to work with physical conditioning for people with functional limitations because of my own situation. I wanted to be an olympic athlete and trained very rigorously. My body couldn't take the stress I was imposing on it, my hip began to degenerate, and this resulted in considerable pain and a noticeable limp. I resolved that this hip problem was not going to stop me and moved into physical training work with the YMCA. Physically limited people were drawn to me because they saw me as a fellow sufferer.

At the Kaslow Center, I work with people to get them started. They have learned to focus on what they can't do rather than on what they can do. I also find that most people have little or no knowledge of how their body moves or which muscles they use for various tasks. Once they have experienced some difficulty with muscle coordination, this lack of knowledge is definitely in the way when they try to reestablish impaired function. As part of our Stress/Stamina program we begin by reawakening various muscles and learning which ones are used to pick up a fork, lift a leg, or tie a shoelace.

Patients often are so afraid they will fail that they focus totally on that fear instead of what they can do to reach some goal. If they fear they will spill a glass of water, rather than concentrating on the fear or the shame that incident might bring to them, I have them work in private. We teach them the individual movements they will need to master in order to pick up a glass and bring it to the lips: reaching the arm out, grasping the cup, lifting the arm, etc. I ask people to practice action by action, rather than jumping to the final goal too quickly.

The patient practices reaching for the cup, picking up the cup, bringing it to the lips, tipping it, then setting it down. Working slowly in private with each step brings confidence from success rather than shame from failure. If one can focus on the muscles used in the action rather than cursing the unsteadiness, improvement begins.

This takes time. Many so-called disabled people have plenty of time and lament that they have so little to do with it. We urge them to get started on simple activities they can practice at home and review with them any problems that they may encounter.

Feelings of shame are the greatest barrier I have to help people overcome. One of the best ways to avoid this shame is to work out games the person can play when no one is watching.

One young woman in her twenties who had multiple sclerosis had difficulty speaking because she felt thick and slow in her facial muscles. She was ashamed of how she sounded and had given up speaking almost altogether. I asked her to get a mirror and make faces at herself: stick out her tongue, wink, open and close her mouth, wrinkle her lips. It was like biofeedback. She could see when she was succeeding and reinforce her own progress. She practiced in solitude and regained the confidence she needed to be more assured in public.

It's as if the body has forgotten how to do things and needs to learn again. This seems particularly true with multiple sclerosis patients and accident cases, both of which involve trauma to the nervous system. It is also true of other disabling conditions, such as stroke.

It is so important for people to be able to perform regular functions, like tying shoelaces, turning door knobs, fastening belt buckles or brassiere clips, using tableware, turning a water faucet on and off. It is incredibly frustrating not to be able to do these everyday things. We focus our efforts and practice on functional tasks until they can be performed effectively.

One patient, a man in his thirties, was experiencing both multiple sclerosis and arthritis. He saw his body as an enemy and was determined to win over it. Every time I watched him move his arms and legs I could see the strain of pain overlaying his weakness and the conflict his viewpoint created. He was desperately "trying" against his own resistance. When he started to reach for an object on a table, his whole shoulder, back, and torso muscle system was braced for his expected failure.

We worked with identifying the muscles he needed to lift something from the table. There were very few in the shoulder and arm. The others could relax and let the few work it out. He did not need to involve his entire body in this small act and struggle with the task.

We began by having him reach out gently, take the corner of a newspaper page between two fingers, then gradually crumple up the whole page until it made a ball in the palm of his hand. These were separate muscle actions that did not need massive effort. He soon learned to approach these movements without the strain of trying. As he regained confidence in his body, his anger subsided. He learned to praise his own success and thank his body for its cooperation rather than blaming it for failure. This greatly eased the difficulty he had experienced with movement and coordination.

Patients who have lost contact with leg and foot muscles have other games they can play. One effective one is to sit in a chair and place a golf ball, small rubber ball, or ping-pong ball beneath one foot. Then, slowly move the foot about, rolling it around on the ball. This gently massages the bottom of the foot and also makes contact with the muscle movements required to move the leg; there is no risk of failure and no weight to bear.

One patient, Marsha, a woman in her mid-thirties with multiple sclerosis, had numbness in her hands and feet and foot drop. She played a game manipulating coins with her fingers, first on a table top, later by twirling them through her fingers like a magician. This rapidly developed fine muscle dexterity in her arms and hands, and it was fun to accomplish without the risk of failure and shame at some more visible public task.

One older woman, in her seventies, loved music. She had become disoriented and had a hard time comprehending conversations, which frustrated her and her daughter. I saw an opportunity to improve both her motor coordination and her listening and attention. I suggested to her daughter that she play dance music with a steady beat and encourage her mother to dance. The woman loved it. The rhythm was calming and directed her attention, the dancing improved her coordination and control. Involvement and movement is frequently more effective than any dramatic medical treatment or drug.

A man in his mid-fifties had been a construction worker and was accustomed to heavy labor and regular association with his hardy, robust fellow workers. When he came to the Center, he had been in a wheelchair with multiple sclerosis for three years and was deeply depressed as a result of his loneliness and inability to move about.

Using mirrors to retrain his facial muscles, crumpling newspapers to get him in touch with small muscles in his arms and hands, and rolling balls with his feet to relearn control of leg muscles, he got moving again. He would set up small wastebaskets around his room. When he had finished rolling up a newspaper ball, he would "shoot baskets" with them. Soon, he progressed to darts and a dart board. When he became confident enough to play with others, he began to spend time at a local club that had a dart board, regaining valuable social contact and self-esteem.

The concept is really the same for the improvement of all chronic dysfunctions. We get people moving—to do something they *can do*—then gradually improve on the range of activity as skills develop. Success and self-confidence are paramount, so people should start in private and try things in public only after they are sure of their abilities.

Don't label yourself by what you can't do. Movement and flexibility are your final goals and they take time and practice.

In addition to my movement and flexibility work, I try to get patients in touch with the heart and lung system and how well they convert oxygen. This is important for everyone, disabled or not.

In the workbook in the following chapter, we explain a simple procedure anyone can follow for measuring this vital capacity. Using the pulse rate as a yardstick, one can chart a "resting" pulse rate and then compare this to a pulse taken after measured amounts of exercise.

Doing this simple exercise teaches one to be aware of the heartbeat indicated by the pulse rate and what it feels like to charge up the cardiovascular system. Everyone should exercise enough to elevate the pulse rate sometime each day, ideally for an increasing period of time up to about 15–20 minutes per day. This is the idea behind jogging and aerobics.

But don't push yourself and feel guilty if you are not doing as well as you "think you should." Exercise should be enjoyed; it ought not to be a boring chore. Begin some exercise you like to do.

Dialogue in Human Concerns

As we have mentioned throughout the book, most patients arriving at the Kaslow Centers have lost self-esteem, feel a loss of control over the destiny of their lives, and have experienced indifference, failure, and disappointment in their interactions with other medical facilities. The resulting anxiety and doubt need to be brought into the open and shared at an honest level. This sharing process is not "psychotherapy" nor are people likely to be told that their problem is all in their head. The purpose of the dialogue is to open up a discussion of the patient's story, to hear out the fears that may have been pent up inside, to clear up any anxieties or apprehensions about the program itself, and to offer some practical and positive skills people can use to identify and deal with stresses in life.

Juliet Sponsel, the Dialogue in Human Concerns counselor, wants to clarify patients' needs, discover what they expect from the Kaslow Program, and provide positive direction and suggestions for attitude clarification.

The process begins with the Self-Awareness Survey, which is reproduced in the workbook. This survey provides an opportunity for the patients to think about a number of questions about themselves and their illnesses. It is important to know how each of us sees personal illness and its effect on life.

Some persons gain unconscious benefits from being chronically ill. Their incapacity brings them attention and caring from people who otherwise may have been indifferent to their needs. If these feelings are present, they can be gently surfaced and discussed. The individual may not be aware of the role this need for attention can play in long-term illness. Although everyone needs some sort of attention, new styles of interaction with others can be learned which can gain the needed attention without the dependency on the illness.

Essentially the dialogue concerns itself with what the patient can see as possible, what is chosen as the vision for the future, what are past abilities that can perhaps be recovered. The program wants to turn "I can't" into "Let's begin." Willingness and persistence are two important qualities for success. The dialogue supports the development of these attitudes.

A Note from Juliet Sponsel,
Dialogue in Human Concerns Counselor
In my experience, many of the patients who come to the center have lost the sense that they can be loved for who they are. They have become identified with their problem and think of themselves as broken and unworthy. This leaves them with a sense of isolation and loneliness. So, I just start loving them. I try to discover their hopes and expectations, their dreads and fears.

Many people have experienced repeated failure and disappointment with other medical centers and doctors. They arrive at the Kaslow Center with either a wide-eyed hope for an immediate cure or an established attitude of skepticism. Neither position is a realistic approach to self-care but suggests to these people that we are here to either provide immediate, miraculous relief or that we should prove we can do something for them. Fortunately, or unfortunately, depending on how one looks at it, we are likely to do neither.

Our aim is to draw out individuals' inner strength and get them moving on their own. A person's sense of control over events in life is central to our success. All our processes here are designed to teach the patient how to gain that sense of control, and perhaps my area of the program is most directly focussed on this issue. I want to discover those seeds of self-worth and zest for life which can be nourished and supported.

It's very important to listen to the story of an illness. Many people are surprised to realize how life events such as job changes, relationship difficulties, money crises, or loss of loved ones seem to coincide with episodes of the illness. One hardly needs to prompt these "coincidences"; they just naturally unravel as the person tells about the illness.

Chelsea spoke earlier about the young woman suffering from chronic depression who was obsessed with her meals and designed her diet as if it were a chemical formula. Her Diet Survey looked like an autobiography, a record of her search for some specific answer to all her problems through nutrition.

When this woman first came in to see me, she was an interesting paradox. She complained of feeling cold and clammy all the time, having no energy or lasting power, and of being too weak to make it through the day. Verbally, she was a torrent of energy. She began with a rapid-fire discussion of her stringent diet regime. Other doctors had told her she was "hypoglycemic" and our tests confirmed wide swings in blood sugar levels during the nonprocessed carbohydrate test.

From her story, I gained information about her that was rather significant. She and her husband had owned their own business, but had lost it four years before and ended up more than $80,000 in debt. They had worked this debt down to less than $15,000, but she had endured four years of pressure from bill collectors, never knowing when the phone rang who would be hounding her. In the middle of all this, her first child had been born. Sometimes when she was trying to care for the baby, the utilities would be turned off for nonpayment of the bills.

She would hide in the house when people she did not know came to the door for fear they were process servers. On top of all this, her mother was an alcoholic and she had to deal from time to time with her mother's erratic actions. Her child was hyperactive and ate alone because his hyperactivity made her too nervous for him to eat with the family. Her husband's failure to give her a financially secure home was an unspoken resentment she had been harboring for four years. She wanted out of her marriage, but could not imagine how she would manage with her young child.

All of this came pouring out without a great deal of prompting. It became quickly clear that this woman was using her physical symptoms as an explanation for her feelings of helplessness about all her emotional distress. She was an acute example of both "pile-it-on" and "double-bind" stress, which was seriously distorting her body's ability to self-regulate. She did not have the skills to relieve these pressures. Being sick allowed her to back away from some of her duties and responsibilities.

In the course of our interviews, she realized she had married her husband to escape an unbearable living situation with her alcoholic mother. She still had expectations of rescuing her mother from her problem, because she had always felt that her health was contingent on her mother's health.

Truth is usually stranger than soap operas. This woman was dealing with all these pressures in the only way she knew how— getting sick and having an excuse to stop and rest. She felt she couldn't discuss her anxieties and fears with her husband because he was bound up in them. She didn't have the power to discuss them with her mother, because she was afraid that doing so would just reopen all the wounds of mistrust and disappointment in their relationship. Driven "inside" by the bill collectors and her fears, she had been holding all this tension in her body *alone* until it finally all burst out in my office. She looked on herself as a victim of her own life.

Just releasing all this pent-up energy changed her appreciably. This relaxation allowed her body to self-regulate more effectively and some of her physical symptoms began to wane. She felt more energetic and more capable of working with her problems.

By the third time we met, she was considering a separate apartment for her and her child, but did not consider a divorce necessary until she had a clearer picture of her relationship with her husband. After all, he had been going through all these stresses and problems just as she had! They both needed some time to regather their energies and assess the future. Her anxieties about her child subsided, hence *so did his hyperactivity!* The child had been confused and upset by her tension and fear.

Her "hypoglycemia" gradually disappeared and her blood sugar normalized. Once the accumulated stresses of her tumultuous life were recognized and accepted, she learned to face them more productively and positively.

This woman had considered herself a failure and was guilt-ridden by her inability to manage her life. Another patient, Brian, was an example of how the drive to succeed and outperform everyone eventually overburdened his body and brought on disease.

Brian was a life insurance salesman who had been the top man in his division three years before, a success in everyone's eyes. He had a large suburban home with an expansive garden he loved. He was an active leader in his church.

He arrived in our office about a year after having been diagnosed as having multiple sclerosis. Much of his left side was nonfunctional and he could walk only with great deliberation and difficulty. Because of his religious background, he had a tendency to think, "Why has God done this to me?"

As our interviews progressed, his need to excel at his work and to achieve perfection surfaced. He had been successful in meeting this need until three years ago, when he was "struck down." His wife had left him. His eating habits became erratic. A fast food devotee, he ate alone and "on the run." His free time was spent at bars to alleviate his loneliness. Eating was only a chore. One and a half years after she left, he began to become ill. He married again six months later to a nurse who could care for him. Shortly thereafter, he had to give up his spacious home and beloved garden because he could no longer care for them.

As we continued to talk, it became more apparent that he considered himself a failure. Since his wife had left, he was punishing himself for failing as a husband. He felt himself unworthy of business success, unworthy of his fine home and garden, and was becoming an emotional and physical cripple who only wanted to be taken care of. The resulting deterioration of his physical abilities confirmed his self-opinion. Once he had labeled himself as a multiple sclerosis victim, his dysfunction forced him to deal with his failure and imperfection.

Brian needed some positive actions he could take to reverse this negative picture of self-worth. We began to work on some exercises he could do to improve his self-confidence and physical capacity.

Brian had been a successful bowler and remembered using visual techniques to improve his scores. Visualization involves the simple process of picturing an activity in your imagination before undertaking it. When bowling, Brian would imagine himself holding the ball, approaching the lane, and releasing the ball just right for a strike. He would practice this in his imagination as he sat on the bench awaiting his turn and would take himself through the mind pictures once again just before he stepped up to bowl. He knew that this technique had improved his bowling skill.

We discussed this technique to improve his left side function. Could he imagine himself walking and running freely? He could picture in his mind those functions that had become difficult, such as walking, working with tableware, climbing stairs, and tying his shoes. Remembering his success with this technique in bowling, he could use it effectively now for more crucial needs. He was put on the total Kaslow Program and the change in diet gave him a running start to getting well.

Brian's new wife came with him to subsequent sessions for Nutritional Counseling and further Dialogues in Human Concerns. Together, we discussed the importance of supporting his improving general state of movement and action and the importance of not overprotecting his condition. As a result of our work together, Brian's persistent nutritional, physical and emotional stress was relieved and he began to move more securely within two weeks.

It is critically important for people to take the time to assess the levels of conflict and stress in their lives and find new ways to work them out.

I find working with people to sustain their self-confidence and provide them with new skills very rewarding. Readers can use the Self-Awareness Survey and the attitude questionnaire in the workbook to explore their own areas of stress and tension.

Frequently, just recognizing them, acknowledging their importance in your life, and talking them over with someone is enough to release their hold on your body and allow your energy to change to a positive direction.

LOOKING BACKWARD:
THE KASLOW PROGRAM REVISITED

Each of the staff members at the Kaslow Center has shared with you the insights and experience gained working with patients at the Center in Santa Barbara. We hope this familiarity with their experiences can give you the motivation and support to try your own "at home" program based on what you have learned in the book so far, and on the workbook which follows in the next chapter.

From the staff experiences and viewpoints, we hope you have obtained an understanding of the very different approach to chronic disease represented by the Kaslow Program. Throughout the book, we have explored this view that our efforts are directed toward rebuilding and revitalizing the body rather than treating disease. Our experience with this program in chronic and degenerative disease supports the validity of this view.

Again, there are five factors, *all under your control*, that appear to be the essential elements in restoring the body's natural capacity for self-regulation and self-healing:

1. Identifying and removing from the diet those foods not tolerated by the body which are causing continuing harassment of stressed tissues (the Metabolic Rejectivity Syndrome).

2. Planning a diet of freshness, variety, and nutritional balance that will provide the needed elements for health.

3. Identifying and relaxing unresolved life stresses, both emotional and physical.

4. Developing body flexibility, movement, and oxygen utilization capacity through exercise.

5. Developing attitudes of self-direction, self-esteem, and well-being based on personal experience of success.

As we have described the several aspects of the Kaslow Program designed to address these five factors, by necessity we have had to separate the activities at the Center into the work done by each staff member and describe each procedure as a separate step. This makes it appear that the several aspects of the program are divided up and that someone might arrive and just try one or two parts of the program and leave the others out.

Such is not the case. All dimensions of the program are interwoven. It is difficult to say just what "heals" someone or which aspect may have been most important. Each member of the staff supports the entire program and sees it as integrated and complete as a total plan.

We say this to encourage you to work with all components of the workbook rather than picking and choosing those which may seem easiest or to your liking on first examination. Give the entire process a try and you may discover some unexpected insights and gains.

Again, we review the factors found to lead to success, as revealed through the survey, taken in Chapter 1, of our successful patients.

- *Motivation* to find a new solution to a seemingly unsolvable problem.

- *Acceptance* of your body as something you can work with, not an enemy to be overcome.

- *Self-knowledge*—an interest in your possibilities, your present situation, and your capacity to change.

- *Sensitivity* to your body and its messages to you, learned through the exercises in Response Diet Testing, Stress/Stamina Balancing, and others. Learn to listen to your body.

- *Persistence*—it takes some time for systemic dysfunctions and chronic problems to develop. Be willing to take the time to turn them around.

Your Doctor's Response

Do not expect an unqualifiedly enthusiastic response from a physician about a program such as this. You may be setting yourself up for a disappointment you need not experience.

Many patients come to Santa Barbara, experience significant change in their problems as a result of the program, then return to their previous physician expecting applause and validation of their success. We wish we could say that this has been a positive experience for many. It has not.

Because of the very different premise on which this program is built, as compared to traditional medicine, many doctors find it a complete mystery and cannot believe what is happening. At times the physician's response is likely to be one of anger or indifference because the patient has sought care elsewhere, especially since that care has proved successful. The frustration and powerlessness felt by patients suffering from chronic and degenerative diseases is also felt by physicians, but they are usually unwilling to admit to it. Hence, when someone finds a successful pathway to return to an effective functional state and good health, the physician may feel as if he or she has been outwitted and defeated.

If your physician becomes angry or seems to reject your willingness to try this kind of program, evaluate whether he or she seems to be more interested in protecting professional control of your situation than in your improving health and welfare.

Fortunately, there are a growing number of physicians who will support these activities and your willingness to take control of your own situation. We hope you have one or can find one.

Remember that there is nothing in this Program that creates unusual risk or danger for you or your body. Everything is under *your control* and can be carried out according to *your plan*. And it's *your* health that you'll be improving.

8

A PERSONAL
WORKBOOK
FOR HEALTH

THROUGHOUT THE BOOK, WE HAVE ENUMERATED THOSE factors that distort the natural self-healing processes in the body, particularly in the chronically ailing body, and we have illustrated that these factors are all influenced by life choices under the control of the individual. Food rejectivity, nutritional imbalance, unresolved stress, lack of physical exercise, and negative attitudes about life and illness are all aspects of life that each of us can become more aware of, assess within the context of our current situation, and change as we see fit.

The purpose of this workbook is threefold:

1. *Information*—to provide you with important self-knowledge to assist you in moving toward and maintaining good health

2. *Activities and Projects*—to offer some practical and interesting opportunities to further your journey

3. *A Journal*—to keep a personal record of your progress and reflect the changes you achieve (the surveys and diary are designed to be used many times over, so it is a good idea to photocopy the appropriate pages or to use a separate sheet of paper for your answers, particularly if this is a library book).

188

The workbook activities are organized according to the aspects of the Kaslow Medical Self-Care Program discussed in the earlier chapters:

- Metabolic Rejectivity and General Nutritional Balance
    Diet Survey
    The Resting Fast
    Response Diet Testing and Diet Planning
    Relaxed Bowel Habits
- Dialogue in Human Concerns
    The Self-Awareness Survey
    The Life Change Index
    Improving the Quality of Personal Interaction
- Stress/Stamina Balancing
    Stress Recognition Exercises
    Meditation and Affirmation
    Progressive Relaxation
    Body Awareness and Movement
    Cardiovascular Fitness
- Planning Your Health Calendar

In each of these activities, we have tried to communicate the essence of the program so that you can discover for yourself a workable pathway to your own health.

Much of this workbook has to do with attitudes, habits, and new life choices. If your previous point of view has been that the future of your health could only determined by physicians and other health care professionals, then many of the directions asked of you here will be new and challenging.

Working with attitudes and changing old habits can be difficult to undertake alone. Everyone needs support and affirmation when new directions are undertaken. It could be useful for you to find one or two family members or friends who would enjoy sharing the journey with you. This sharing can make the experience more enjoyable and will also serve to keep the process going.

Select people to share with you who will not criticize you or the process but will explore its possibilities with you. People who have a habit of telling you what your situation is and what you should do about it without listening to you will probably make poor traveling companions. Choose people that you like to be with and who make you feel good, rather than people who criticize you or make you feel incompetent.

Work with these activities according to a plan, but don't feel pressured to do everything at once. Take your time. You didn't develop chronic problems in 24 hours and it is unlikely that you can change your body into a healthy and marvelous machine by the end of the week. Be patient with yourself and expect an occasional setback.

YOUR ATTITUDES AND THEIR ATTITUDES

Your attitude about your health possibilities is the most important factor. However, we realize that it can be difficult to plow through the barriers that other people's attitudes can put in your path and still feel a sense of freedom and accomplishment. If people around you are not supporting your journey to health, don't confront or blame them. Instead, minimize your interaction with them in your new journey.

Assess the professionals, physicians, and counselors you see for health care and advice. If it seems that they are not listening to you but are just telling you what to do without regard to your needs, feelings, and participation, that's probably exactly what is happening. If they make absolute statements about who you are, what is happening to you, or what may happen to you in the future—without any consideration for the impact these statements have on you—then they may be of little service to you in the long run.

Instead of these professionals, seek those who are willing to take the time to listen to your questions and hear about your needs. These people may be harder to find, but it is worth the effort. *There is no point in continuing to do what does not work,* even if you have been told there is no other course available.

Discourage professionals, friends, and visitors who want to tell you how your problem reminds them of their problem, or someone else's problem. Instead, talk about interesting things people are doing or thinking about doing. Plan a positive future. If no one around you is talking about or doing interesting things, you might try some new environments some of the time.

If the people around you dwell on your problem, feel sorry for you, and make you feel less than a full person, arrange some more cheerful surroundings for at least some of your day or regularly throughout the week.

Professional Dependency

Many of us have been taught to feel that circumstances in life are determined by events and opinions of others beyond our control. As you look at the following descriptions of possible situations, think about the factors that will be likely to *initiate change* in your situation and where control over those factors lies. Each situation described lists a different combination of your opinions and the opinions of others.

Situation 1:

I think my life circumstances are under the control of others or outside forces. I feel there is nothing I can do until others tell me what to do and how to do it.

Others, who act with authority and apparent certainty, tell me there is nothing that can be done to change my situation. I defer to them.

Since you feel powerless to act without instructions from others, and others tell you nothing can be done, then no action will emerge from this situation and you will continue to feel powerless and helpless.

Situation 2:

I think my situation is hopeless and there is little possibility of improvement. I don't listen to what others say because they don't understand my predicament.

Others tell me there are ways I can find improvement and new possibilities and they bring me suggestions and ideas. I don't think it's worth the effort.

Even though others have hopes for a better future in this situation, your resistance to that possibility will most likely prevent any progress. In this situation, your personal attitude is apparently the only barrier to your moving from helplessness to action.

Situation 3:

I think there may be some ways I can change my situation for the better, but I'm not confident of that. I'm willing to look around and check out new possibilities.

Others, who act with authority and apparent certainty, tell me nothing can be done to change my situation and I should live with it.

Improvement is possible here. It will take a great deal of courage and self-confidence to proceed in the face of the apparent indifference of others to your interests and needs.

Situation 4:

I think there are ways to change my situation for the better and I'm willing to continue to check out new possibilities, even if some don't seem to work.

Others support me in my inquiry into possibilities and are patient with the process, recognizing that I may not encounter success in every endeavor.

With the support and encouragement of others, a great deal of progress is likely in this situation.

As you review these situations, realize that the primary determinant of likely change is what *you think*, not what others think or do. Without the support of others the task is more difficult, but you are the primary director of the course of action. With the support of others, a great deal of positive movement can occur. Again, the key factor is what *you think can happen.*

METABOLIC REJECTIVITY AND GENERAL NUTRITIONAL BALANCE

Increased nutritional awareness offers you three ways to support your body's self-healing and self-regulation processes.

1. Identification of foods your body is rejecting, thereby stimulating your immune system and harassing stressed tissues. Elimination of these foods from your diet will stop this degenerative process.

2. Reduction of or elimination from your diet of substances that are not supporting your body (additives, colorings, chemicals, refined foods), because they either stress the metabolic process or fail to provide essential elements.

3. Creation of a balanced and nutritious meal plan that will give your body the essential elements it needs for action energy, tissue building and maintenance, and effective self-regulation.

The activities provided to increase your nutritional awareness and assist you in food planning are the Diet Survey, the Resting Fast, Response Diet Testing, Diet Planning, and Relaxed Bowel Habits.

The Diet Survey

The Diet Survey focuses your attention on an overview of your eating habits and the content of your diet. Most people evolve eating habits over a long period without a direct awareness of how they have made these choices, what total diet picture these choices create, and what cumulative effect on health the diet they have chosen may produce.

The following survey lists a number of foods in various categories and asks you to indicate how frequently you eat these foods. Mark your responses on photocopies that will serve as worksheets.

Sit down and consider how often you eat each food and check the appropriate space. Include everything you take in during coffee breaks, between-meal snacks, and late evening refrigerator raids. There is no need to cover up or make excuses. You are the only person evaluating this process, so be honest with yourself. If you feel the need to hide something, then look at the reasons for eating the foods that trigger this response. You are apparently already aware of your distrust of their value to your health.

If there are foods in your regular diet not listed on our survey, just enter them in the appropriate category in the extra spaces. You are the only one interpreting the survey and you'll know why you put in the extra entries.

KASLOW MEDICAL SELF-CARE DIET SURVEY

EGGS AND DAIRY PRODUCTS	NEVER	OCCASIONALLY	ONCE A WEEK	2-3/WEEK	4-6/WEEK	ONCE A DAY	2-3/DAY	4 OR MORE/DAY
MILK, RAW								
MILK, PASTEURIZED								
MILK 2% OR LOW FAT								
MILK, RECONSTITUTED, DRY								
MILK, CHOCOLATE								
BUTTERMILK OR KEFIR								
CHEESE, CHEDDAR OR AMERICAN								
CHEESE, COTTAGE								
CHEESE, OTHER								
YOGHURT								
BUTTER, SWEET CREAM								
BUTTER, OTHER								
MARGARINE								
ICE CREAM								
SHERBET								
EGGS, FRIED OR SCRAMBLED								
EGGS, POACHED								
EGGS, BOILED								
EGGS, RAW								
EGG WHITES								
PROTEIN DRINKS, MILK BASE								

BEVERAGES (Nondairy)	NEVER	OCCASIONALLY	ONCE A WEEK	2-3/WEEK	4-6 WEEK	ONCE A DAY	2-3/DAY	4 OR MORE/DAY
COFFEE, NATURAL								
COFFEE, DECAFFEINATED								
TEA, ORDINARY								
TEA, ROSE HIP OR OTHER HERB								
ORANGE JUICE, NATURAL 6 oz. or less								
ORANGE JUICE, NATURAL over 6 oz.								
ORANGE JUICE, IMITATION								
GRAPE JUICE								
GRAPEFRUIT JUICE								
OTHER CITRUS JUICES								
OTHER NON-CITRUS FRUIT JUICES: Please list below and indicate usage.								
1.								
2.								
VEGETABLE JUICES, FRESH								
VEGETABLE JUICES, CANNED								
BEER								
MIXED ALCOHOLIC DRINKS								
SOFT DRINKS								
SOFT DRINKS, DIET								
GINGERALE								
DRINKING WATER, TAP								
DRINKING WATER, Distilled or Spring								
PROTEIN DRINKS, JUICE BASE								

DIET SURVEY, CON'T

MEATS	NEVER	OCCASIONALLY	ONCE A WEEK	2-3/WEEK	4-6/WEEK	ONCE A DAY	2-3 A DAY	4 OR MORE/DAY
LEAN BEEF CUTS (Steak, Roast, etc.)								
BEEF (Cut purchased and ground)								
BEEF, GROUND (Preground at store or served in restaurant)								
LIVER (BEEF, CALF, OR CHICKEN)								
HAM								
PORK ROAST, CHOPS, ETC.								
BACON								
SAUSAGE								
TUNA								
LOBSTER								
SARDINES								
FISH CAKES Halibut, Trout, Catfish, etc.								
OYSTERS, SHRIMP (Boiled)								
OYSTERS, SHRIMP (Fried)								
OTHER SEAFOOD (Boiled, Baked, Fried) Please list below and mark the times eaten.								
1.								
2.								
CHICKEN (Fried)								
CHICKEN (Broiled or Baked)								
PREPARED FOODS								
TACOS, ENCHILADAS								
PIZZA OR LASAGNA								
HAMBURGERS								
HOT DOGS								
COLD CUTS, Sandwiches								

DIET SURVEY, CON'T

GRAIN FOODS	NEVER	OCCASIONALLY	ONCE A WEEK	2-3 WEEK	4-6 WEEK	ONCE A DAY	2-3 DAY	4 OR MORE DAY	
CEREALS. DRY. BOXED SINGLE GRAIN									
CEREALS. GRANOLA TYPE									
WHEAT GERM									
OATS. COOKED									
GRITS									
OTHER CEREALS, COOKED									
BREAD, WHITE									
BREAD, NATURAL WHEAT OR RYE									
BREAD, SOY									
BREAD, CORN									
MULTI-GRAIN BREAD									
BREAD, SPROUT									
PANCAKES OR WAFFLES									
MUFFINS, WHEAT OR CORN									
ROLLS, PLAIN OR BUNS									
ROLLS, SWEET									
CAKE OR PIE									
COOKIES									
CRACKERS, SODA OR SNACK									
CRACKERS, GRAHAM									
DOUGHNUTS OR PASTRIES									
MACARONI OR NOODLES									
PRETZELS									
RICE, WHITE									
RICE, WHOLE, BROWN									

FLOWER, FRUIT, AND SEED VEGETABLES	NEVER	OCCASIONALLY	ONCE A WEEK	2-3/WEEK	4-6/WEEK	ONCE A DAY	2-3/DAY	4 OR MORE/DAY
BEANS, LENTIS (Dried, Baked)								
BEANS, LENTILS, BLACKEYED PEAS (Dried, Boiled)								
BEANS, GREEN OR LIMA								
PEAS, GREEN								
SOYBEANS								
SQUASH								
TOMATOES								
BROCCOLI OR CAULIFLOWER								
CORN								
CUCUMBERS								
EGGPLANT OR OKRA								
MUSHROOMS								
PUMPKIN								
PEPPERS								
ARTICHOKES								
MISCELLANEOUS								
SOUP								
NUTS								
PEANUT BUTTER								
SUNFLOWER SEEDS								
GELATIN								
JELLIES, SYRUP								
CHIPS, CORN OR POTATO								
CANDY								
CHOCOLATE (Candy, Cookies, Cake, etc.)								

DIET SURVEY, CON'T

ROOTS AND TUBERS	NEVER	OCCASIONALLY	ONCE A WEEK	2-3/WEEK	4-6/WEEK	ONCE A DAY	2-3/DAY	4 OR MORE/DAY
BEETS								
CARROTS								
PARSNIPS								
POTATOES (Boiled, Baked)								
POTATOES (Fried)								
RADISHES								
RUTABAGAS								
TURNIPS								
ONIONS (Fresh or in cooked dishes)								
ONIONS (Fried)								

LEAF AND STEM VEGETABLES

	NEVER	OCCASIONALLY	ONCE A WEEK	2-3/WEEK	4-6/WEEK	ONCE A DAY	2-3/DAY	4 OR MORE/DAY
ENDIVE, PARSLEY, CHIVES, CRESS								
GREENS, BEET, TURNIP, MUSTARD CHARD, KALE (Cooked)								
CABBAGE								
SAUERKRAUT								
CELERY								
LETTUCE								
BRUSSELS SPROUTS								
SPINACH								
ASPARAGUS								
RHUBARB								
SPROUTS, BEAN								

DIET SURVEY, CON'T

FRUITS	NEVER	OCCASIONALLY	ONCE A WEEK	2-3/WEEK	4-6/WEEK	ONCE A DAY	2-3/DAY	4 OR MORE/DAY
CITRUS FRUITS								
APPLES, PEARS (Whole or Stewed)								
APPLESAUCE								
PRUNES, PLUMS								
FIGS, DATES								
GRAPES, RAISINS								
BANANAS, AVOCADOS								
CRANBERRIES, WHOLE OR SAUCE								
BLUEBERRIES								
BERRIES, OTHER								
PEACHES, APRICOTS								
CHERRIES								
MELONS								

DIET SURVEY, CON'T

MEAL FREQUENCY	NEVER	OCCASIONALLY	ONCE A WEEK	2-3/WEEK	4-6/WEEK	ONCE A DAY	2-3/DAY	4 OR MORE/DAY
BREAKFAST								
LUNCH								
SUPPER								
SNACKS								

LIST PRESENT MEDICATIONS AND FREQUENCY	NEVER	LESS THAN ONCE A DAY	ONCE A DAY	TWICE A DAY	THREE DAY	MORE THAN THREE DAY		
1.								
2.								
3.								
4.								
5.								
6.								
7.								
8.								
9.								
10.								

After you have completed the Diet Survey, ask yourself the following questions.

Content

- Am I choosing foods from several of the food groups, or do my selections seem to concentrate in just a few?
- How much of my food is fresh or frozen compared to prepared and packaged foods or fast foods from restaurants?
- Based on the essential food elements listed in Chapter 5, is my diet offering me a variety of these elements, or am I missing some of them?
- Do my choices lean toward fats and fried foods?
- How much sugar am I eating in foods, in drinks, and in packaged foods (see Table 5.1)?
- Are my snacks nutritious or mostly sugar or stimulants?

Habit

- Do I eat the same foods for certain meals almost every day?
- How frequently do I repeat the foods I choose?
- How many of the foods listed on the survey do I eat regularly?
- How many of the foods listed on the survey do I not eat at all?
- Do these items I never choose seem more nutritionally desirable, about the same, or less nutritionally desirable than my current choices?

Take a brief imaginary trip, picturing the steps you go through in meal planning, shopping, and meal preparation. Think about how much of this process has evolved out of convenience and habit, and how much of it is related to providing your body with the nutrients it needs.

Do you want to change your eating habits so that if you did a survey of this type several months from now, the results would look very different to you? After we have explained the Response

Diet Testing, suggestions will be given for planning and preparing meals based on variety, foods your body likes, and assurance of including the elements your body needs.

In general, you probably already have a sense that diets concentrated around certain kinds of foods may not nourish your body. If you eat mostly meats, fats, and fried foods, your diet lacks balance. Some sugar is almost inevitable if one is buying supermarket foods, but diets with a high concentration of sugared foods, sweets, and sugar in coffee will most likely overload the liver/pancreas metabolic system for regulating sugar in the body. Diets consisting mostly of packaged and refined foods will contain additives and chemicals unwanted by the body and will tend not to contain essential minerals and vitamins required by the body.

Once you have looked at an honest diet survey, you will probably have an intuitive sense of what you need to do to change your diet to a more balanced situation. Listen to that intuitive sense. After you have completed the Response Diet Testing, this sense will be greatly improved and validated. It can become the basis for your new nutritional program.

The Resting Fast

The Response Diet Testing that follows requires an ability to be aware of the body's responses to the ingestion of individual foods. In order to gain a reliable assessment of these responses, you must start with a relatively quiet system. The way your system functions now is the result of its responses to your current food habits; hence we need to give it a break before we begin the Response Diet Testing. Therefore, we precede the testing period with a 48-hour distilled water fast.

During this fasting period, the self-regulation systems in your body will tend to reset themselves at more natural levels, because they will not be stressed by any foods. Once they have done this, your responses to foods will provide a more accurate gauge of your body's likes and dislikes.

As you are fasting, drink plenty of distilled water, at least, if not more than, eight full glasses each day. This will move liquid through to clear your system.

We use distilled water (available at most grocery stores) because local water supplies may contain chemicals and additives that will stress the body. The bottled mineral waters are also not recommended since their mineral content may affect the testing.

If you are feeling weak and run down, you may be afraid to try the fast, fearing it may further weaken you. Perhaps you feel you must eat every day as an expression of your determination to keep going. We applaud your determination; however, the eating process may be the factor that is causing your weakness and lack of energy. A pause to reevaluate will most likely improve, rather than worsen, your situation. Many of the patients at the Center in Santa Barbara express feelings of great relief and symptom amelioration during fasting!

If you are feeling weak and fatigued, don't try to fast and also maintain a busy schedule of activities. Take a break and rest as you fast, allowing your body to relax and regain its internal balance. Even is you have a reasonable level of energy as you begin the fast, don't push your body with continuing or heavy physical exertion during a fasting period. Take it easy.

Should you experience some anxiety or stress during the fasting period, take yourself through the progressive relaxation process described later in the workbook.

The fasting period is a good time during which to make your plans for the Response Diet Testing. Look over the test foods list in the next section and choose the ones you will test, planning your first five-day cycle.

Response Diet Testing and Diet Planning

The purpose of the Response Diet Testing is to discover and remove from your diet any foods that cause significant physical, emotional, or psychological reactions when you eat them. A side benefit of the testing process will be a markedly increased awareness of your physical, emotional, and psychological states throughout the day and how they can be affected by foods, as well as by other events and situations.

The Response Diet Test consists of (1) removing from your diet plans high-risk, processed, and refined foods; (2) selecting test foods from the recommended list; (3) preparing and eating these foods one at a time per meal, four meals per day; and (4) keeping a diary of your responses to these foods.

General Rules for the Test

1. Precede the testing period with a 48-hour distilled water fast, as previously described.

2. Do not use any condiments, sauces, or spices during the Response Diet Test period. Season foods only with sea salt and sweet creamery butter. _OLIVE OIL

3. Do not test "high-risk" foods; i.e., milk and dairy products, gluten grains (wheat, oats, rye, or barley)—use brown rice, millet, potato, or soy flour as substitutes. Among the patient population suffering chronic diseases who have undertaken Response Diet Testing, these high-risk foods are the most frequently found to be rejected. Hence, we do not include them in the early testing period, thereby reducing the risk of a strong adverse reaction. This gives your body time to readjust without severe stress.

4. Do not eat any sugar, refined flour products, processed foods containing additives or preservatives, or chocolate during the test period. After the testing we recommend that you give up these items altogether.

5. Do not drink coffee, soft drinks, or teas during the test period. Use distilled water for drinking and cooking.

6. If you are a smoker, give up smoking during the test. Once your body is rebalanced as a result, you may find that your need to smoke has diminished or disappeared.

7. Do not take any vitamins or minerals as supplements on the one-food-at-a-meal testing days. If you feel the need for them, take them only on the variety days when you are eating foods that have tested suitable to your metabolic state.

8. Do not drink alcoholic beverages, wine, or beer during the testing period. Sweet fruit juices should also be avoided.

PROTEINS

— SARDINES - IN WATER

1. Beans, Soy
2. Beans, Pinto
3. Beans, Navy
4. Beans, Lima
5. Beef, Ground
6. Beef, Roast
7. Beef, Steak
8. Chicken
9. Cod
10. Cornish Hen
11. Eggs
12. Halibut
13. Lamb
14. Liver, Beef
15. Liver, Chicken
16. Red Snapper
17. Salmon
18. Sand Dabs
19. Sea Bass
20. Sole
21. Swordfish
22. Trout
23. Turkey
24. Veal

③

for 3 DAYS

VEGETABLES

1. Asparagus
2. Alfalfa Sprouts
3. Bean Sprouts
4. Beets
5. Broccoli
6. Brussels Sprouts
7. Cabbage
8. Carrots
9. Cauliflower
10. Celery
11. Cucumbers
12. Egg Plant

13. Green Beans
14. Jicama
15. Lettuce
16. Mushrooms
17. Mustard Greens
18. Onions
19. Parsley
20. Peas
21. Radishes
22. Rhubarb
23. Rutabagas
24. Scallions
25. Spinach
26. Squash
27. Sweet Potato
28. Swiss Chard
29. Tomatoes
30. Turnips
31. Yams
32. Zucchini

SPECIAL NUTRIENTS
(COMPLEX CARBOHYDRATES)

②

1. Corn, on Cob or Popped
2. Rice Cakes
3. Natural Brown Rice
4. Millet
5. Potato, Boiled or Baked
6. Corn Meal

RAW NUTS AND SEEDS (UNSALTED)

①

1. Filberts
2. Walnuts
3. Brazils
4. Cashews   *ALMONDS*
5. Peanuts
6. Pecans
7. Sunflower Seeds
8. Sesame Seeds

9. Keep your diary faithfully. If you are aware of a strongly
   distorting event (a disturbing phone call shortly after
   eating, a traffic ticket, or the like) take that into account
   in assessing your response to foods. You may want to
   retest any food that produced an adverse reaction if there
   is a possibility that some outside event might have upset
   you. You will develop a trust in your intuitive sense of
   the origin of the upset.

The Test Food List

The list of foods on p. 206 is a fairly comprehensive selection
of foods, excepting those ruled out above. If you have some additional foods you want to add to the test list, do so in the appropriate column, being sure not to include the high-risk processed
or refined foods.

Because fruit and sugar sources of carbohydrate have been
removed during this testing period, we have highlighted the
complex carbohydrates so that you will be sure to include adequate energy foods in the test plan. Peas are also a high carbohydrate food among the vegetables. Also, different kinds of
lettuce or cabbage as well as different fish can be considered as
"different" when preparing your test food lists.

Select 12 foods from the lists on p. 206. Include three proteins, two complex carbohydrates, one of the nuts and seeds, and
complete your choice with vegetables.

During the first 3 days of the test period, on completion
of your 48-hour fast, prepare 4 moderate size meals every day.
Each meal will consist of only 1 food chosen from your list of
12, prepared with sea salt and sweet creamery butter only as
flavorings.

Table 8.1

INDIVIDUAL FOOD TEST EXAMPLE

EXAMPLE	FIRST DAY	SECOND DAY	THIRD DAY
Meal 1	Eggs	Peas	Millet
Meal 2	Zucchini	Peanuts	Celery
Meal 3	Lettuce	Chicken	Carrots
Meal 4	Sweet Potato	Potato	Navy Beans

On completion of this cycle, on the fourth and fifth days, prepare four small meals each day consisting of combinations of small portions of these same twelve foods, something like a Chinese restaurant meal in which you have small portions of several different foods on your plate.

Do not include in this fourth and fifth day combination any foods that caused adverse reactions during individual testing. These foods should be removed from all further testing and diet

Table 8.2

COMBINATION MEALS EXAMPLE

EXAMPLE	FOURTH DAY	FIFTH DAY
Meal 1	Eggs	another variation
	Peas	
	Carrots	of the list for the
	Celery	
	Sweet Potato	fourth day,
	Chicken	
		making new
Meal 2	Millet	
	Navy Beans	combinations
	Potato	
	Peanuts	
	Lettuce	
	Zucchini	
Meal 3	Eggs	
	Peas	
	Carrots	
	Potato	
	Peanuts	
	Lettuce	
Meal 4	Chicken	
	Sweet Potato	
	Celery	
	Zucchini	
	Millet	
	Navy Beans	

planning for a number of months. Retest these nontolerated foods at a later date when you have achieved a level of optimum well-being.

Prior to the sixth day, select 12 additional foods from the lists, again choosing 3 proteins, 2 complex carbohydrates, 1 nut/seed, and filling in the rest with vegetables. On the sixth, seventh, and eighth days, return to eating only 1 food per meal, using these 12 *new foods*, testing them as you did on the first 3 days, 1 food per meal and 4 meals daily. On the ninth and tenth day, you can again prepare combination meals, but you will now have 24 foods (minus the rejected foods) to choose from.

You can continue through these five-day cycles until you have tested all the foods on the list. To make things come out even, you may have to include some foods you have already tested in the later cycles. If there were some doubtful outcomes, or if you have favorites, you can repeat them.

How to Keep Your Diary

Make about 12 copies of the *Response Diet Testing Diary* that follows, 1 for each day of 4 testing cycles, each lasting 3 days. As you begin each testing day, enter the date and the foods to be tested in the appropriate spaces on a sheet for that date. As you sit down to each meal, enter the time at which you ate that food. Then, set a timer or make a mental note to check yourself and *make entries* in the diary at one-half hour, one hour, and two hours from the time you began eating.

When entering your responses, avoid general statements like "feel bad" or "OK." Look for signs and behaviors that are more specific. Here is a check list.

ABDOMEN

Belching
Bloated
Cramps
Diarrhea
Gas—rumbling
Hyperacidity

Nausea
Thirst
Vomiting

EARS

Itching
Blocked
Ringing

Ache
Hearing loss
Acute sensitivity to sound

EYES

Itch, burn
Tears
Heavy and tired
Blurred vision
Spots or flashes
Acute sensitivity
Vision loss
Double vision

JOINTS

Ache
Stiff
Swelling
Heat
Sharp pain

MOODS AND EMOTIONS

Confusion
Depression
Negativity
Listless/withdrawn
Anxious
Fearsome/panic
Irritable/angry
Alert/talkative
Hyperactive
Intoxicated/silly

MUSCLES

Jerky
Weak
Spasms
Ache

NOSE

Sneezing
Stuffy
Nasal Drip
Itch
Sinus accumulation

GENERAL FEELINGS

Dizzy, loss of balance
Faint
Chilly or cold
Hot flashes
Fatigue
Stimulated and active
Tense and restless
Heaviness
Irritable or hyperkinetic
Crying

HEAD

Headache, mild
Pressure
Throbbing
Migraine

HEART/LUNGS/CHEST

Cough
Wheezing
Pressure
Starved for air
Rapid breathing
Chest pain
Throbbing or rapid pulse

PERCEPTION/ORIENTATION

Dreamlike or sleepy
Momentary loss of reality
Disorientation

Hallucination
Paranoid/fear of attack
Wandering
Inability to focus attention
Insomnia

SKIN

Itch—indicate site
Perspiring
Heat
Hives
Flush
Lose tone and color/ghostly
Cold clammy hands or feet

SPEECH

Sluggish or sleepy

Stammer or word repeating
Can't organize words
Reading/speaking errors

THROAT/MOUTH

Hoarse
Bad taste
Sore throat
Tender gums
Acid taste
Sore tongue
Choking or tight throat
Teeth hurt
Postnasal drip

On the fourth and fifth days, and on subsequent combination days, use a new response diary sheet. List for each of the four "foods" the combinations you have selected. It is not as likely that you will obtain a strong undesirable response from a *combination* of foods already shown to be acceptable, but it may happen. You can discover by the process of elimination those combinations of foods that do not go well together.

RESPONSE DIET TESTING DIARY

Date:

Food #1 (name of food):

Eaten at (time):

Response at one-half hour:

Response at one hour:

Response at two hours:

General comments:

Food #2:

Eaten at:

Response at one-half hour:

Response at one hour:

Response at two hours:

General comments:

212

Food #3:

Eaten at:

Response at one-half hour:

Response at one hour:

Response at two hours:

General comments:

Food #4:

Eaten at:

Response at one-half hour:

Response at one hour:

Response at two hours:

General comments:

After you have proceeded through four or more cycles of this food testing, you will have built up a list of accepted foods and nontolerated foods. You will also have experienced the preparation of foods in the Chinese-style combinations. This is the recommended routine for you to continue indefinitely, preparing foods from your acceptable list and making up combination meals.

Later, you can:

1. Retest dairy foods, grains, and fruits. Plan a one-food meal every now and then when you are feeling good, balanced, and healthy. Try one of the foods from the above three groups to assess your body responses as you did during the earlier testing cycles.

   It is not wise to set up a retest schedule of three days made up entirely of these foods. Should several of them cause severe reactions, you may have a setback that is unnecessary.

2. Reintroduce condiments, sauces, and spices. You should do this gradually and watch your responses; by now your finely tuned sense of your body's requirements will identify those that should not be used.

3. Reintroduce teas, herbs, juices. Again, introduce these gradually, one at a time, and assess your response.

4. Enjoy a meal out in a restaurant or as a guest. Select carefully. We realize there can be great temptation to indulge yourself and think that "since I'm feeling so great" it won't matter what you eat. Remember, you are *feeling great because of what you eat*. You already know from experience that you are sensitive to foods—in the euphoria of feeling good, we ask you to remember.

General Suggestions

Eat variety. Check the lists of foods in Chapter 5 that indicate the vitamin and mineral content of various foods. Plan your combination meals around a variety of these foods to assure intake of each of the essential elements. If you want a more comprehensive study of the issue, consult Chapter 15, "How to Choose

Your Own Nourishment" from Roger Williams's *The Wonderful World Within You.*

Eat fresh. Try to obtain fresh foods and eat them as fresh as you can. As we've said many times, avoid packaged foods.

Moderation is a good guide. Don't do a lot of anything, but a little of many things.

Eat lightly. Heavy, concentrated meals will weigh you down. Salads, vegetables, eggs, and fish can give you all the basic foods you need. If you like beef, eat smaller portions. Pastas and sauces are enjoyable once in a while, but again, moderation is the key.

Stay with it. You will begin to feel better when you follow this food plan. It's almost a natural response to become over-confident and forget the role food plays in your health. Don't let yourself slide back into illness and impaired function after you've learned the keys to staying healthy and feeling vital.

After all the complex material you've read or heard about regarding nutrition, you're likely to say, "Is this simple program all there is?" Yes. It's as simple as knowing what your body wants and can metabolize and then forming your own plan to meet its needs. Nothing else is needed! *

Relaxed Bowel Habits

One of the frequent results of the American diet and life-style is constipation. When compiling information for this book, it was interesting to note few index listings for "bowel." However, there were always some under "constipation." This is but another example of this society's preoccupation with problems rather than with an understanding of basic functions.

When we focus on problems, we think in terms of fixing them. Hence, the widespread promotion of laxatives, bulk-pro-ducing cereals, and the like. Constipation is a signal from the body that one of the natural self-regulation systems is not work-ing well. Fixing the constipation does not necessarily solve the problem. We must start by identifying those factors that may be distorting the body's natural capacity to process solid wastes. These are:

---

*Please see The 8 Mini-Food Meal Program update on page 265 for our revised—and simplified—food plan.

Lack of adequate liquid. The lower intestine withdraws liquids from the food remnants remaining after digestion and assimilation in order to "recycle" them in the body. Through the process of osmosis, it takes from the liquid nutrients what it needs for use elsewhere. If total liquid intake is low, the result will be dry and hard stools. During the food testing, drink plenty of water. Later, as you have tested various liquids, include plenty in your daily routine. We do not recommend a large daily intake of citrus juices because of their high content of simple carbohydrates. However, fresh vegetable juices are excellent liquids.

Diets high in meats, low in fiber. Meats leave less bulk residue in the intestine than do fiber foods (leafy stem vegetables, some grains).

Deficiencies in B vitamins. Diets deficient in B vitamins deprive the body of important nutrients necessary for effective body function. Check the foods listed in Chapter 5.

Lack of exercise. All body functions require movement and stimulation. Body activity fosters intestinal movement, thus maintaining the intestinal system pliable and flexible. Regular exercise helps your body establish good bowel function.

Stress, worry, unexpected changes. If you are "holding back" on an important decision, "waiting" until you arrive at a more comfortable location, "holding in" worries about work or home situations, or accustoming yourself to strange surroundings, your body tends to tense up. Bowel elimination is chiefly a relaxation process, so learning to relax will greatly benefit bowel function.

Straining to achieve a bowel movement can be counterproductive. Instead, as you read about the progressive relaxation exercises, discussed later in the workbook, learn to relax the muscles especially in the abdomen and buttocks. *Relaxation* of these muscles is more likely to produce a movement than pushing and straining, actions likely to lead to hemorrhoids.

We've heard for years that it is "normal" to have one bowel movement each day. More recently, we've discovered that the concept of what is normal should give way to individuality, as we actually exist in nature. Some people have more than one movement daily, others daily, some less frequently. Our suggestion is to become sensitive to, and listen to, your body and accommodate its signals.

DIALOGUE IN HUMAN CONCERNS

In the metabolic rejectivity response food testing and in general nutrition planning, we now know that foods and food habits affect health in ways not previously recognized. Because of foods rejected by the body, deficiencies of essential elements result, such as trace minerals and vitamins. Over a long period of time, rejection creates a continuous stress on the natural self-regulation systems of the body designed to maintain health. By learning more about the signals from the body telling us what it "likes" and "does not like," we can alter our food choices and their reactions. These changes lead to a greater awareness of factors that affect health. This ultimately results in reestablishment of normal function, eliminating dysfunction and physical limitations to open the pathway to health and well-being in a natural way.

This same process applies to other aspects of life in addition to nutrition. Habits built over the years can cause continuing low-level stress without our recognizing what is happening. Our life patterns develop gradually, choices are made, situations emerge, but we have not learned to take the time to assess and reflect. Stress becomes accepted and is looked on as a normal state in our life pattern and then becomes a regular routine without recognition of its possible consequences.

The Dialogue in Human Concerns has an objective similar to the Response Diet Testing. The exercises and activities in this section will confront you with a number of questions. For some, dealing with these questions is like testing foods. Some questions you will like, some you will want to reject, some will seem trivial and uninteresting.

Our lives have many facets. Our work, our living situation, our families and its relationships, how we spend our leisure time, and who we look to for assistance and support all can provide emotional nourishment, or worry, or stress, or indifference. Frequently, we are not aware of our responses to the different factors in the life situation. The exercises in this section are designed to bring these factors to your attention. At your leisure and without anyone's judging or measuring you, you can ask yourself the questions and assess your answers. There are no right or wrong answers, just your personal reflections about issues in your life. Which are important to you, which are unimportant, which are stressful and worrisome? Which would you like to discuss?

Because a number of these issues are raised in the Dialogue in Human Concerns, physical exercises for managing your stress by relaxing your mind and body will be provided in the Stress/ Stamina Balancing section. Once you are aware of the stressful factors in your life it becomes possible to change them and above all to personally choose new actions.

Self-Awareness Survey

The purpose of this survey is to raise a series of questions about your life, your interests, and your sense of self. The survey is a guided tour through those aspects of life that are the usual sources of discomfort and stress.

Not all the issues will be important to you. Some may seem of little importance or pointless. However, to someone else those issues might spark a special insight or raise a significant question. Hence, we have tried to include as many viable alternatives as we have derived from our experience with hundreds of people seeking the sources of their stress and discomfort. So, you need not question why something is included that seems obvious or trivial. Just go on to the next question and look for the ones you find interesting.

Generally, the questions fall into three categories: interesting (want to think about it a bit), uninteresting (so what?), and provoking (want to avoid, distressing, wish that hadn't been asked). Note the interesting ones and the provoking ones on a piece of paper. After reviewing the entire survey, you can come back to these issues and give them some thought, and at times it helps to share your feelings about them with someone.

The interesting ones may lead to insights about some choices you have made in the past that you now realize may have caused your stress. Look at these situations with the view that they may lead to new possibilities and choices.

The provocative ones most probably represent areas of your life you would rather avoid and not have to deal with. These are sources of continuing stress to be recognized and surfaced. As you are more willing to explore these issues, they may move into the "interesting" category, provide some valuable insights, and open up new choices and possibilities, relieving the *stress of avoidance.*

Perhaps the best way to work with this survey is to make a photocopy of the survey pages so that you can write your responses on the working copy. This way, you can keep a record of your responses for later review. (You may want to repeat the survey in several months to see what changes have occurred in your responses. You may be surprised!) If you prefer, you can mentally answer the questions and simply note the items of interest and provocative issues. We do recommend that you spend some time after completion of the survey reflecting on those questions raised in your mind by the exercise. That is what the survey is designed to generate.

SELF-AWARENESS SURVEY

Date:

Full name as given at birth:

Name you use now:

What name do you really like to be called?

Do some people call you by a name you don't like?

Have you ever changed your name?

Make a note of the circumstances involved in changing your name:

Would you prefer another name?   If so, what would you like?

Do you like your present age?

What would you consider to be an ideal age?

What are some of the special qualities someone your age might have that someone another age might not enjoy?

Do you enjoy being the sex you are?

220

Is being the sex you are   ____ important to you
                             ____ a primary issue in your sense
                             of self
                             ____ unimportant to you

Have you ever wondered what it would be like to be a person
of the opposite sex?

Do you have any fears about qualities you exhibit which
might be considered to be those of the opposite sex?

Have you recently   ____ gained weight   ____ lost weight?

Do you consider your weight   ____ far above ideal
                              ____ somewhat more than
                              you like
                              ____ acceptable
                              ____ ideal
                              ____ somewhat lighter than
                              you like
                              ____ far below ideal

Do you feel your weight situation is beyond your personal
control?

Your father's name:

Is your father still living?

If so, does he live ____ in your home ____ nearby
____ far away

Allow a picture of your father to come to mind. Briefly describe him and the situation you pictured.

How do (did) you feel when interacting with your father? (check all that apply)
____ great ____ OK ____ confused ____ childlike
____ nurtured ____ sad ____ creative ____ enthusiastic
____ powerless ____ angry ____ rejected ____ loved
____ other (describe)

Your mother's name:

Is your mother still living?

If so, does she live ____ in your home ____ nearby
____ far away

Allow a picture of your mother to come to mind. Briefly describe her and the situation you pictured.

How do (did) you feel when interacting with your mother? (check all that apply)
____ great ____ OK ____ confused ____ childlike
____ nurtured ____ sad ____ creative ____ enthusiastic
____ powerless ____ angry ____ rejected ____ loved
____ other (describe)

Names of brothers and sisters (or others important to your childhood):

Are you close to these relatives now? Do you see them regularly or correspond?

Describe in a few honest words how you feel about your sense of family with your childhood family (that is, as compared to the family in which you may now be a parent or grandparent).

Who would you say was the most important person (or two or three persons) in your childhood?

What one statement could you make about the contribution of each of these persons to your life?

Was someone in your childhood family seriously ill?

Do you remember illness, doctors, and concern for health in your early years, either for yourself or for other family members?

What does that memory mean to you now?

If you have children, list their names:

Make a brief statement about the qualities you like especially in each child:

Make a brief statement about some aspect of each child that particularly upsets or distresses you:

Consider some aspect of your relationship with your children you would like to improve:

If you are working, describe briefly how you see your work role:

When you leave for work in the morning, are you:
_____ looking forward to the day?
_____ planning the day with some concern, but confident of your ability to manage the job?
_____ confused about how you will complete the day?
_____ worried about projects and your personal progress?
_____ dragging yourself to a job you find unpleasant?

Are your answers to the above consistent, or do they swing back and forth based on (a) current tasks and their stage of completion, or (b) current state of your relationships with coworkers?

Is your current work interesting?

How do you feel about your progress with your present employer?

List a few people with whom you now work whom you enjoy and feel supported by:

List a few people with whom you now work that cause you to worry or to become upset:

List those aspects of your present work that occupy your mind when you are away from work:

What might you do to change the situations you have listed above that you spend time worrying about?

Do you feel adequately paid for the work you do?

Can you discuss issues of pay, workload, and working conditions with your supervisor or employer(s) in a forthright way?

Is your work schedule, or commuting schedule, stressful or tiring?

If you are not working because of an illness or dysfunction, how do you feel about the situation? (check any that apply)
_____ I am bored and would like to get back to work
_____ I am glad to get away from a job I could not stand
_____ I feel like a victim of my problem and can't seem to get going again
_____ I think I would like to start a different kind of work (Make up your own reply that most clearly states how you feel about your situation.)

Make a brief list of the people who are "closest" to you (do not include your children unless they are adults and interact with you as adults).

Make a statement or two about each of these persons discussing some aspect of each you truly appreciate. Have you shared your appreciation recently?

Is there some aspect of your relationship with any of these people about which you worry? Can you share this issue with the person and perhaps resolve it?

Is there some subject about which you find it difficult to speak with each or any of these people?

Is it difficult to talk about any of these issues: sex, money, loneliness, habits that irritate you, values, power?

When you talk with the people close to you, are you usually: (check any that apply)

____ sharing ideas and feelings	____ reminiscing
____ seeking information	____ worrying about problems
____ complaining	____ planning
____ criticizing	____ doing projects together
____ giving instructions	____ passing the time
____ receiving instructions	____ other (describe)

Is there someone with whom you feel you can share your innermost fears and secrets?

Are you hiding any worries or fears that you don't want *anyone* to know?

Are you currently in a relationship offering you expression of your sexuality?

Are you satisfied with this relationship?

Is the relationship such that you can talk about interests and needs?

Do you daydream about sexual interests you feel are unsatisfied?

Do you feel guilty about these interests or these daydreams?

Check any of the following in which you participate:

	DAILY	SEMI-WEEKLY	WEEKLY	SOMETIMES
running/jogging	___	___	___	___
walking	___	___	___	___
swimming	___	___	___	___
bowling	___	___	___	___
golf	___	___	___	___
calisthenics	___	___	___	___
dancing	___	___	___	___
softball/baseball	___	___	___	___
physical labor	___	___	___	___
weight lifting	___	___	___	___
bicycling	___	___	___	___
tennis	___	___	___	___
other (describe)	___	___	___	___

Do you consider that you have a regular exercise program?

In your work, or in your daily routine, are you:
____ sitting most of the time?
____ moving about occasionally?
____ mildly active?
____ on your feet most of the time, but not doing physical work?
____ doing regular physical work?
____ doing strenuous physical work?

If you have some physical limitations as a result of illness or injury, do you think of yourself as disabled or unable to regain mobility?

Does this make you sad or angry?

If you could regain mobility and action, are there things you would like to do?

Check problems you experience which may be related to lack of movement:
____ occasional pounding heart
____ muscle soreness after exercise
____ general fatigue
____ tired on awakening
____ bowel irregularity
____ tension and irritability
____ occasional shortness of breath
____ avoidance of participation in activities

Check activities in which you participate:

	DAILY	SEMI-WEEKLY	WEEKLY	SOMETIMES	NOT DOING, BUT WOULD LIKE TO
social clubs	____	____	____	____	____
educational classes	____	____	____	____	____
plays, theater	____	____	____	____	____
Bible or study groups	____	____	____	____	____
movies	____	____	____	____	____
playing cards	____	____	____	____	____
dancing	____	____	____	____	____
painting	____	____	____	____	____
writing	____	____	____	____	____
crafts and hobbies	____	____	____	____	____
watching TV	____	____	____	____	____
shopping	____	____	____	____	____
travel	____	____	____	____	____
reading	____	____	____	____	____
gardening	____	____	____	____	____
camping	____	____	____	____	____
hiking	____	____	____	____	____
bowling	____	____	____	____	____
swimming	____	____	____	____	____
golf	____	____	____	____	____
tennis	____	____	____	____	____
fishing	____	____	____	____	____
hunting	____	____	____	____	____
volunteer service	____	____	____	____	____
visiting friends	____	____	____	____	____
other (describe)	____	____	____	____	____

How many hours do you sleep each night?

Do you usually fall asleep easily or are you frequently restless?

Do you take any medications to help you relax or sleep?

If so, how long have you been taking these medications?

Do you frequently want to sleep in the daytime or take naps?

Do you feel as though you get enough sleep? Too much?

Do you awaken refreshed in the morning?

Do you recall your dreams?

Are they pleasant or do they disturb you?

Stand nude in front of a large mirror. Look at your entire body.

Does this embarrass you?

What parts of your body do you appreciate?

What parts do you feel unhappy about? Is this because they are failing, do not look right, or don't fit together to make a pleasing appearance to you?

Do you consider yourself to be attractive or potentially attractive?

Did you feel good or bad about your body as a child?

Consider some things you can change about your body:
weight, capacity for movement, general tone and appearance.
What would you like to change?

Consider some things about your body you may be unhappy
with but cannot change: face shape, general bone structure,
features, height. Can you accept these as a part of yourself
without blame or a sense of disappointment?

Are there hair styles, clothing styles, or general toning up
processes you can use to make you feel better about your
physical self and its presentation to the world?

Describe your current living environment: (check all that
apply, add others to suit)

____ in a home	____ parent, small children	____ spacious
____ in an apartment	____ parent, older children	____ crowded
____ in a mobile home	____ grandparent/ relative	____ private room
____ other:	____ older child	____ share room with spouse/ partner
	____ sharing with friends	____ share room with sibling/ relative
	____ sharing with relatives	____ other:
	____ other:	

What do you like about your present living environment?

What would you like to change about this environment?

Do you have adequate access to needs, such as shopping, transportation, parks, work, schools, etc., which you regularly want to utilize?

List a few things in your living or work space that brighten your day, i.e., pictures, flowers, plants, colors, books, etc.

Are there things you would like to add to your living or work space that would brighten the space?

If you were to do three things to brighten your living or work space, what would you do?

Do you feel relaxed and comfortable in your living and/or work space?

If not, what are the factors that seem to diminish your feelings of relaxation and comfort?

Are there repetitive noises that nag at you and put you on edge, for example, dogs barking, heavy street traffic, machines running, squeaky refrigerator, leaky faucets?

If you are working:
   How long does it take you to get to work?

   How do you travel?

   Do you consider your commute to be a chore and a burden?

Are there noises, flickering lights, persistent telephone calls, or other nuisance factors that disturb your work?

Are there gases, chemicals, noisy machines, or other factors near your work that, although accepted as routine, seem to lurk under the surface of your awareness as bothersome and stressful?

Do you get upset or frustrated when you drive a car in traffic?

Do you have to drive in traffic almost every day?

Are you comfortable in your car?

Do you consider yourself a calm driver?

Have you had a traffic accident within the last year?

Do you receive traffic citations?   ____ regularly
____ frequently   ____ rarely

Do you wear your seat belts?

Check one or write your own:
____ I'm busy doing the things I enjoy
____ I never seem to have enough time
____ I'm sometimes bored and restless
____ I don't seem to notice the clock, time just goes by
____ other:

Using a calendar of the current month, recall your past week.
Mark the approximate time you spent: (there may be
overlapping items)

____ working to earn a living
____ taking care of yourself (relaxing, being with friends
       and loved ones)
____ doing errands
____ enjoying sports
____ sleeping
____ watching TV
____ commuting
____ doing busywork to pass time
____ daydreaming
____ procrastinating
____ reading or enjoying a hobby
____ preparing meals
____ eating
____ being creative
____ other:

If you could design an ideal week of activities such as those
listed above or others of your choice, what time allocations
would you imagine?

What do you consider the most creative project or activity
you have accomplished in your life?

Is this a type of activity you still enjoy?

Have you done something within the last month or so that
you consider creative? (planted a garden, drawn a picture,
written a story or a poem, built something)

What type of project gives you that true glow of completion and satisfaction?

Are you now engaged in such a project?

Do you feel generally financially secure?

How do you feel when you sit down to pay bills?
____ worried about making ends meet
____ satisfied that you can pay them all
____ concerned for the future
____ doing a routine task
____ financially independent
____ other:

Do you feel your income is adequate to meet your needs?

Do you feel you manage money well?

Do you end up getting most of the things you need and want?

Do you get into differences of opinion with others about money matters?

Do you worry about money issues frequently?

Do you see some possible ways to resolve your money worries?

Consider a typical week in your life. Make an entry next to each of the following words indicating approximately the number of hours you spend experiencing that feeling each week. Don't worry about adding up the time and being accurate, just give yourself a picture of the allocation of time. If you think of your work time as very separate from your personal time, do a separate review of each and see how they compare.

____ active	____ sad	____ frustrated	____ fruitful
____ lonely	____ relaxed	____ blessed	____ rebellious
____ upset	____ productive	____ depressed	____ meek
____ angry	____ worried	____ confused	____ powerless
____ excited	____ over-	____ anxious	____ controlled
____ fatigued	loaded	____ enjoying	____ tense
____ pleased	____ satisfied	____ enthusi-	____ day-
____ powerful	____ busy	astic	dreaming
	____ dis-	____ behind	____ other:
	organized	schedule	

Check the words that describe you:

____ lonely	____ heavy	____ friendly	____ sexy
____ intelligent	____ cranky	____ cautious	____ independent
____ secure	____ desirable	____ disabled	____ aspiring
____ humorous	____ bored	____ colorful	____ broken
____ frightened	____ healthy	____ capable	____ insightful
____ bright	____ pleasant	____ depressed	____ plain
____ confused	____ limited	____ funny	____ outgoing
____ tall	____ light	____ caring	____ persistent
____ unloved	____ clever	____ happy	____ bad
____ hopeful	____ muddled	____ hiding	____ able
____ adept	____ open	____ progressive	____ dependent
____ verbal	____ attractive	____ plodding	____ neat
____ sensitive	____ anxious	____ pudgy	
____ protective	____ serious	____ improving	
____ creative	____ bungling	____ worried	
____ sad	____ intuitive	____ slim	

The Significant Life Change Index

Frequently, the effects of stressful events significant to our sense of well-being can accumulate without our recognition of their impact on us. In Chapter 4 we described the Life Change Index and how points accumulated on that tally might indicate predisposition to serious illness.

Such an index is not very precise for each individual because events of high stress to one person may go unnoticed by another. Therefore, we're going to ask you to create your own stressful event index.

Taking a brief journey through your memory, recall the past eighteen months. Make a note of any significant event that shook you up or changed your sense of well-being, such as an auto accident, traffic tickets, onset of illness, divorce, marriage, child leaving home—any life event that seems relevant.

Now, think of something that would truly disturb you, such as the death of someone close, and give that event a value of 100. In comparison to that event, give the other significant events that you remember within the last eighteen months a point value.

How many events do you list? Were there several serious events of more than 50 points? What is your total point count?

Realize that an accumulation of serious events (not all necessarily "bad") can build up stress without your being aware of it, changing your view of yourself and your capacity to handle your life. Knowing how stressful your life has been can relieve some of your anxiety about your capacity to cope. If you have experienced a number of exceptional events or setbacks within the last year and a half, recognize their impact on your life and give yourself a chance to relax and recover balance. In the Stress/ Stamina Balancing Section, you learn mind-focusing and progressive relaxation techniques to assist you.

Improving the Quality of Personal Interaction

Illness and dysfunction can prove very frustrating and difficult. One of the results of this frustration can be that you interact with others in a way that drives people away and furthers your frustration. As the nutrition, relaxation, and exercise patterns in your life change, so will your attitudes and feelings. Many of your irritabilities and frustrations may wane, and you will feel more like being with and sharing with others. However, your relationship patterns are also habits like nutrition and exercise. People have certain expectations about how you are likely to act. Give them time to appreciate the new you.

One suggestion for changing the quality of your interaction with others is to avoid blame statements, statements that blame others for actions that upset you:

You just don't care for me.   You always forget to . . .
You never . . .   You didn't . . .
You always . . .   You're just . . .
Why don't you ever . . .

You may have resented it when people made such statements to you. Avoid perpetrating that conflict yourself by making statements expressing what you think and feel rather than attributing blame or failure to the other person.

It is also productive to avoid direct commands and control statements:

Bring me . . .
If you don't . . . , I will . . .
You should . . .
If you keep that up, I'll . . .

People resent these approaches, sometimes without revealing it, and will eventually avoid or resist those who use them. Instead, make simple declarative statements about your needs and feelings, without whining or pleading:

I feel lonely when everyone goes off without saying goodbye.

I sometimes get upset if I am not included in group decisions.

Since my activities have become limited, I need more time to just sit and talk with someone so I'll feel included in what is going on.

I don't understand what is happening to me and that frightens me. Since we all seem to be upset by that, let's talk about it rather than withdraw and become anxious.

There are no judgments of others in these statements, just information about what is happening and how you feel about it. People can respond to such statements without having to defend a position.

When people who live together or work together start defending a personal position, real dialogue stops and stress and anxiety begin. In order to make such statements clearly, each of us needs to take a moment and assess what is really going on inside. Then we can say what we want to say rather than blurt out an angry accusation.

Remember that people around you may be uncomfortable with changes in you and don't know how to talk about it. They really shouldn't be blamed for their discomfort. If they are, the walls you both build will be hard to knock down. Bring discomfort out into the open.

Taking New Action

A tree that it takes both arms to encircle grew from a tiny rootlet. A many storied building is built by placing one brick upon another. A journey of three thousand miles is begun by taking a single step.

LAO-TZU
Philosopher of the sixth century B.C.

Out of the exercises in the Dialogue in Human Concerns section, you may have identified issues of interest, stresses you had not been aware of, aspects which upset you, and situations you would like to change.

Throughout the book, we have discussed that our first and immediate response to illness is to try to fix it. Generally medical practice uses this approach. To change our thinking on this issue, throughout the book we have spoken of the *natural healing wisdom within each of us!* Now that you have recognized these stresses and issues, you may feel that you must "do something" right away to fix them or change them. However, an important factor is that once you have recognized these issues, they have lost some of their power. The unknown issues are the ones that wear us down the most. The issues in which we feel trapped and powerless come next. We have surfaced some of the unknown ones, and, throughout, we have given you possibilities for action in areas you may have previously thought beyond your control.

In the following section, Stress/Stamina Balancing, we offer a number of relaxation, mind-focusing and meditation techniques. If you establish these techniques as essential in your daily routine, your view of the issues that cause stress in your life will change. We cannot predict how you may decide to resolve or change each issue, but we do know from experience that relaxation and meditation will reveal new answers and possibilities to you from your inner wisdom.

STRESS/STAMINA BALANCING

Stress is a series of measurable physiological responses within the body. When an event takes place that surprises or upsets you, your heart rate increases ("I saw this car coming at us and my heart just raced."), your breathing becomes rapid and shallow ("The phone rang and I could hardly catch my breath."), your blood pressure rises ("I was so angry I thought I'd explode."), and your muscles tense ("I just wanted to get up and run out of there.").

This response is your body's natural preparation for action in the threat of danger. Your automatic response to an upsetting and threatening situation or an unanticipated event is to prepare for direct action or immediate flight. This flight/fight response has been built into your body by millenia of evolutionary experience.

Stress becomes a health issue when events from the past retain these physiological responses in the body long after the situation has passed. Without being aware we are doing so, we "worry" or continue to think about past stress events. At times, based on previous experience, we conjure up possible future, threatening, events. When we do this, the body responds by maintaining a continuum of flight/fight readiness, even though there may be no immediate action to take.

While the body is in this readiness state, many of its normal maintenance systems are idling at a "ready fire" state in order to keep energy readily available for immediate action. Thus, when we maintain this "ready fire" stress "on hold" for a prolonged period, the healing of damaged tissue is postponed and replacement of recycled cells, as well as the usual health-maintaining processes, may be short-changed. In the long run, the body shifts from its normal functional state, and the setting for chronic disease is firmly established.

However, just as stress is a measurable physiological response, so is relaxation. Relaxation allows the body to react in opposition to stress: slower heart rate, slower, steadier breathing rate, lower blood pressure, and relaxed muscles. We have known that we can slow down our breathing rate at will, but it was not seen until recently that we can voluntarily slow the heart rate, lower the blood pressure, and relax specific muscles. The following exercises will teach you how to achieve these parts of relaxation.

Regular practice of relaxation shifts the body and the mind to reset the many self-regulation systems to normal levels. Once this is accomplished, many body functions can return to the natural state of self-healing the body inherently possesses. If you practice the relaxation procedures discussed below regularly, new responses will emerge from your thoughts and actions. Decisions made while relaxed seem more assured, confident, and more lasting than decisions made under stress.

Stress Recognition Exercises

Body Stress

How are you sitting right now? Are you comfortable in your chair? Are there any aches or tightness/tension in muscles as a result of how you are positioned? The first stress recognition exercise is a simple one. Stop occasionally during the day and assess your posture, any symptoms/signals from the body, and your general feeling of comfort or discomfort.

When you are driving a car for a considerable period of time, focus your attention on the comfort or discomfort of your posture and muscle tensions. If you are working at a desk or table, or performing some task at work, periodically check your awareness of posture and any muscle tensions. "Look at" your body from time to time. Arrange to take breaks, inhale deeply a few times, do a few stretches of all body muscles. If driving long distances, stop occasionally and walk about and do a few body muscle stretches. Your body will respond greatly to the change in physical constraints and the minirest period. '

Later in the progressive relaxation section, we explore further additional ways to become more aware of retained stress in the body and how to release it.

Mind Stress

Many of us worry too much. We mentally tell ourselves stories, have long and continuing conversations in our heads, and become frightened about upcoming events or past situations. This chatter in our brains is usually centered around self-doubt. "Should I have? If only I could have, why didn't I? How will they think of me? Will I ever be able to?" etc. This endless mind activity affects our bodies, creating countless actions and reactions throughout the day as these worries are processed.

Catch yourself doing this. For just a few days, keep a notebook handy and jot down a remark or two about the issues that seem to keep your mind running: unpaid bills, a project at work, difficulty in a personal or business relationship, a stressful past event, and so on. (If you run out of issues your mind has been considering, refer to the Self-Awareness Survey in the preceding section!) Then, when you have a moment to yourself, sit down and make a short summary of these self-concerns, further asking yourself:

- What is happening in the situation I am worrying about?

- Are there certain actions I could take to change the situation so I need not spend so much worry on it?

- Which of these actions seems reasonable?

- Am I willing to take that action? Do I need to take any action at all? Will the whole situation work out on its own?

- Is there any way that my worrying is going to change the situation?

If you can think out possibilities and courses of action to resolve the issue, rather than filling yourself with self-doubt, fault finding (of yourself as well as others), and blame placing, much of this brain chatter can be replaced with more productive thoughts. Remember, problem solving takes place when the mind has dismissed the blocking effect of self-doubt.

One of the methods to quiet this chatter is meditation, which we discuss shortly. Another productive tool is the use of affirmations. Affirmations are simple statements of positive actions or goals which you repeat over and over on a regular, ritualized basis to direct the flow of your thoughts. They are usually "I" statements you write yourself which reaffirm your worth and capacity to achieve your aims. Here are some examples:

- Today I am capable of doing everything I need to do now.
- I know I can love and be loved.
- I can be aware of my own needs and discover how to meet them.
- I can learn from the past without blaming.
- I can make a contribution to those around me by listening and caring and by doing what I can to help.
- If I will let it, the world will assist me when I need help.

Sit down and think for a few moments about how you would like to be and how you would like the world to interpret you. See if you can write just a few simple statements of your feelings in a positive, forthright way. If you prefer, find an inspiring book you enjoy and draw some appropriate phrases from the book. Be sure the statements are in the first person, so that your sense is that of making statements about yourself and your feelings. The quotations might have to be changed slightly to meet this requirement.

Make time for yourself at the beginning of each day, or at intervals throughout the day, to take a few moments and quietly repeat these statements. When you find yourself drifting into your worry chatter, realize this and shift your attention to your chosen affirmations.

You may be surprised at the energy you may have during the day just from the simple process of *shifting* your mind from the depressing negatives to the energizing positives.

Meditation

To meditate, interpreted literally, means to bring to the center. Meditation is a skill or technique for centering and quieting activity of the mind. Practicing meditation is a way to quiet the busy voices of your mind, discover the truer sense of self, and allow this more relaxed, sensible self to interact with the present events in your life in place of your former anxious, worried self.

Because the current American interest in meditation evolved from the teachings of Eastern mystics, some people fear it, looking at meditation as a form of worship or religious practice. Meditation can be both of these but need not be either.

Although religious leaders and some other teachers give the impression that learning to meditate is some mysterious process requiring special, or even secret, instruction, it is actually an easily explained process anyone can undertake. Everyone practices a process similar to meditation frequently. When you are daydreaming or "lost in your thoughts," you are engaged in a process very similar to meditation. During these times you can disengage from the active, task-oriented thought process and gradually drift off into an uncluttered different form of thinking and feeling.

Meditation is a voluntary, purposeful, and organized form of thinking, enabling you to be in charge of that thinking rather than drifting off and finding yourself at the whim of your daydreaming.

Meditation is based on two primary activities: directing the pace of your physical activities through adjustments of your breathing, and directing the focus of attention in your mind by setting up and limiting your sensory experiences. Generally we don't pay much attention to our breathing. The body goes on taking in and expelling air as part of its routine function. The rapidity of our breathing is controlled by level of physical activity. When we run or climb stairs, we breathe faster and more deeply. When we sit or lie down, our breathing returns to normal. In meditation, the exercise is designed for you to breathe more slowly than normal. This slows down most of the processes of the body and produces a level of relaxation.

Meditation then organizes mind activity through control of sensory input.

Seeing: staring at a mandala (a circular symbol, such as a rose window in a church, a target, or a circular painting in which figures radiate out from a prominent center), a light, a candle, or a beautiful object.

Hearing: repeating over and over a brief phrase or word, known as a mantra, or listening to drum beats, music or chants. Group chanting is a common meditative practice.

Touching: using prayer beads, small smooth stones, or holding other objects.

Smelling: burning incense, fragrant candles, or using fragrant oils.

Tasting: the sacramental use of certain wines and foods has been practiced in many religious ceremonies, so that a context of quiet attention can serve as a meditative focus.

The purpose of these rituals is to capture the activities of the senses and diminish conflicting input from other sensory stimuli and thereby reduce random mind activity.

A Meditation Ritual

1. Find a comfortable space in which you can be quiet and uninterrupted for a short time each day. Early in the day, mid-afternoon, or both are ideal times. Twenty to thirty minutes are ample for each session.

2. Arrange yourself comfortably. Sitting in a supportive chair with sidearms and a firm back is good. Some people like to lie on the floor with appropriate cushions for support.

3. Arrange your visual environment. Some like to meditate with eyes closed, others with eyes open. If you prefer eyes open, then select something on which to focus your vision: a candle, a mandala, a flower, or the like. It is usually unproductive to choose a painting, photograph, or detailed object, since these bring ideas and content into the mind that get in the way of meditating.

If you prefer eyes closed, the visual environment is less important and yet may be significant. Beauty is an inherent part

of life. Even before closing your eyes, having pleasant surroundings, such as flowers or artistic arrangements within your view,
sets a mood that filters into the depths of the mind.

4. Choose your form of ritualization. Using the sensory
ideas we have been discussing, design some ritual for yourself
that will engage and capture your attention. Slow breathing and
chanting may be satisfactory for some, others may like a pleasant
rhythm or soft music as background for meditation. Sometimes
starting with music can be helpful. The selection criteria are a
slow, peaceful rhythm, quiet melodies, and a consistent mood.
Readings with stirring passages or many shifts in rhythm or mood
are not recommended. Some appropriate selections: "Air on the
G String" from the Suite in D by J. S. Bach; "The Kanon in D"
by Johann Pachelbel; "Meditation" from the opera *Thais* by Jules
Massenet; "Pavane" from *Requiem* by Gabriel Faure. Some suggested mantras or chants to be repeated over and over in a continuing tone: "I am able to be alive"; "I am loved and loving."
A resonant sound, such as o-o-o-o-ou-ou-ou-ou-u-u-u-u-m-m-m-m-m
or, a brief phrase of your own choosing. If you like candles and
incense, use them and make a ritual of preparing your space for
the quiet time. Look forward to meditation as a preferred time
of your day.

5. Get ready. Arrange your music, your environment, and
your ritual plan. Arrange yourself in your chair or on the floor
as you have chosen. It is best if your arms and legs are not
crossed and your arms are resting easily at your sides with the
palms up. Sitting in the Eastern lotus posture with your legs
crossed is not required to achieve successful meditation.

Start by breathing regularly and deeply. Count slowly to
three as you breathe in, hold one count, then count slowly to
three as you breathe out, hold one count, breathe in to three
counts, and so on. Focus your attention on your breathing and
get a sense of how the breath feels in your body. Feel the air
filling your body from the lower torso upward, rather than just
in the rib cage. When you breathe out, feel your body relax and
let the air continue to flow out until the body wants to start a
new cycle. None of this should be forced. Just concentrate on
your quiet, pleasant, and easy breathing.

6. Once you have achieved a sense of relaxed awareness

of your breathing, begin your selected ritual: your chant, focusing on the candle, or whatever you have designed.

Don't begin meditation with a lot of expectations, based on what others have told you should happen or on what others reported happened for them. This is your experience alone and you are not meditating to live up to someone's idea of how it should be done or what should be experienced. Just allow your mind and your awareness to focus on your ritual.

If thoughts or worries come through your mind, don't blame yourself for failure or struggle with them. Just watch them go by without engaging them. When you first begin, this may seem troublesome. Your mind may be overactive and all sorts of issues, ideas, and events may parade by. Take a "so what?" attitude and watch them drift away. Don't be hard on yourself or measure your progress all the time. Just let your mind drift through space while you stare at your candle, or repeat your chant, or listen to your music. With your slow, easy breathing, you find the quiet space in time and accept it joyfully.

7. Be consistent. Schedule your quiet time each day, or regularly during the week, and stay with it. Don't expect miraculous things to happen. Just allow yourself to enjoy the ritual of being quiet on a regular basis.

Eventually you will find a more relaxed attitude toward events in your life. Things that bothered you before may seem less urgent and easier to handle. Events will appear to flow more smoothly around you. Symptoms of unrelieved stress and body dysfunction diminish.

If you have difficulty getting started and need some support, here are a couple of suggestions. Write Cognetics, Inc., P.O. Box 592, Saratoga, CA 95070, and ask for information on the cassette tapes they have to "meditate by." The use of a prepared tape that guides you into a meditative ritual can be helpful in the beginning. There are also two good books on meditation available: *How to Meditate: A Guide to Self-Discovery* by Lawrence LeShan, and *The Second Centering Book* by Gay Hendricks and Thomas Roberts.

Progressive Relaxation

Unrecognized and retained stress in the body is the cause of much pain and muscular dysfunction. In addition, as we have mentioned before, this unrelieved stress can distort the self-regulation systems, affecting digestion, tissue maintenance, cell rebuilding, and other important health-maintaining processes.

Progressive relaxation is a specific ritual designed to (1) create a greater awareness of the stress state of each muscle system in the body and, (2) develop a period of deep physical relaxation for all the major muscle systems. During these periods of deep relaxation, the body has an opportunity to rest, reset the self-regulation systems, and restore more complete functional, natural homeostasis.

Since your awareness is focused during this relaxation process, it is essentially a form of meditation. In addition, it is a learning process about the several muscle systems in the body. As you proceed with the exercise through the various areas of the body, you become more familiar with how your body feels. Places in the body which are painful, lack a sense of contact, or of awareness become more evident. You also learn that by relaxing these areas of pain and stress you experience a pleasant effect on these sensations. These simple techniques can frequently relieve headaches, muscle spasms, and other aches and pains.

The entire progressive relaxation process, even taken quite slowly, takes only fifteen to twenty minutes. Be willing to take longer; don't rush. This could be the most important time of your day. As both a meditation and relaxation exercise, your newly acquired habit can accomplish significant changes in (1) your personal attitude toward your body and your awareness of its function; (2) the flexibility and relaxation of the various muscle systems; and (3) reduction of tensions which can cause headaches, muscle spasms, and gradual dysfunction.

This is a simple yet effective process, which you can do at times of your own choosing. It requires no equipment, no trip to someone's office or gym. And, it feels great!

Progressive Relaxation Exercise

1. Arrange a comfortable sitting position (in a big, comfortable chair with supportive arms) or lying position (on the floor on your back with cushions to support your head, your elbows, and your knees) to relieve any pressure or tension on the entire muscle system.

2. Take a few moments to quiet yourself, resting and breathing easily.

3. Begin to breathe slowly, three counts in, hold one, three counts out, hold one, and so forth, in a continuing cycle.

4. As you breathe in, whisper or think, "I am," as you breathe out, say "relaxed." As you say, "I am" while breathing in, imagine energy from all the world filling your body to replace the tensions as they flow out! As you breathe out and say, "relaxed," imagine the tensions and stresses of your body flowing out with the expelled breath.

5. After you have repeated the "I am relaxed" cycle several times, relish the softer, easier feeling of your body as you continue with a few cycles of deep breathing. Feel how warm and heavy your body feels against the chair or cushions.

6. Focus your awareness on the muscles of your feet. As you breathe in to three counts, tense these muscles, focusing your attention only in the feet. Don't tense up your whole leg and lower body, just your feet, with as little movement of the leg muscles as possible. It may take some practice to isolate each set of muscles. Some connective muscles in the legs will always be involved when tensing the feet, of course. Hold the tension in your feet on the fourth "holding" count, then expel your breath rapidly, saying *aaaahhhh* out loud as you breathe out. Simultaneously, let go of the tension in the foot muscles.

(If you want to take the time, you can work with individual feet, leg, arm muscles, alternating from one side to the other. This will allow an even greater awareness of each area of your body. We describe in what follows the process working with both sides at once.)

7. Flow through another cycle of breathing, three counts in, hold, three counts out, hold, just relishing the warmth and relaxation in your feet, moving the muscles lightly and feeling the freedom. Say to yourself during this cycle, "My feet are warm and relaxed."

8. Move your awareness to your lower leg and ankle. As you breathe in for three counts, tense these muscles, hold the one count, then as you release your breath, *aaaahhhh*, let go of the muscle tension. Move through the extra cycle, enjoying the relaxed warmth and easy movement, saying to yourself, "My legs and ankles are warm and relaxed."

9. Move your awareness to your upper legs and knees. Repeat the breathing, tensing, holding, and letting go cycle. On the extra cycle, say, "My thighs and knees are warm and relaxed."

10. Move your awareness to your hips, buttocks, and lower back. Repeat the breathing, tensing, holding, letting go cycle with these muscles. Enjoy the extra cycle, saying, "My hips and buttocks are warm and relaxed."

11. Move your awareness to your hands and fingers. As you breathe in to the three counts, make a fist, clamping your fingers into as tight a ball as you can. When you release after holding the fourth count, allow your hands to fall open, palms up, on your lap or on the cushions. Enjoy the extra cycle, saying, "My hands are warm and relaxed."

12. Move your awareness to your forearms and wrists. Again use the fist exercise, but focus your attention on your forearms instead of your hands. Do the breathing, tensing, holding, letting go cycle. Enjoy the extra cycle, saying, "My forearms and wrists are warm and relaxed."

13. Move your awareness to your upper arms and elbows. As you breathe in, make your biceps bulge. Then, as you release, drop your arms in a relaxed position. Enjoy the extra cycle: "My arms feel warm and relaxed."

14. Move your awareness to your abdominal and stomach muscles. As you breathe in, tense this area as if you were doing a sit-up, or expected to be punched in the stomach. Then, let go, relax on the expelling of breath and say, "My abdomen feels warm and relaxed," as you enjoy the extra cycle.

15. Move your awareness to your upper chest, ribs, and collarbone area. As you breathe in, lift your rib cage high in an exaggerated puffing of your chest. Then, as you let go, let your chest fall as you expel your breath. Say, "My chest feels warm and relaxed," as you enjoy the extra cycle.

16. Move your awareness to your shoulders and upper back. As you breathe in, lift your shoulders up toward your ears as high as you can. Then, on letting go, let your shoulders drop and droop, with your arms falling into a floppy position at your sides. As you enjoy the extra breathing cycle, say, "My shoulders feel warm and relaxed."

17. Move your awareness to your jaw and neck. As you breathe in, grit your teeth and clench your jaw tightly closed. Then, as you let go, let your jaw drop down loose onto your chest as your head and neck fall forward (if you are sitting up). As you are enjoying the extra cycle, say, "My neck and jaw feel warm and relaxed."

18. Move your awareness to the muscles of your face. As you breathe in, compress all your facial muscles, wrinkling your nose, squinting your eyes, pursing your mouth, as if you were pushing your whole face forward. Then, as you let go, aaaahhhh, again drop your jaw and allow all the facial muscles to go slack. On the extra cycle say, "My face feels warm and relaxed."

19. At the end of this entire sequence, follow through with about ten additional cycles, enjoying the feeling of deep relaxation and saying to yourself, "I am warm and relaxed."

Try It Now. Reread this section and get a sense of the flow of the process. Then, make yourself comfortable somewhere and go through the exercise. Take your time. It may feel a little awkward the first few times. If you stay with it, you can learn to truly enjoy the warmth and relaxation your body may be discovering for the first time in a long time. Relish the relaxation.

If you feel blocked, or feel the need for more specific guidance, write Cognetics, Inc., P.O. Box 592, Saratoga, CA 95070 and ask for a list of relaxation cassettes. There are some very good ones that will guide you through sequences similar to those we have described, giving you instructions as you go.

Body Awareness and Movement

Every individual, at any age and in any condition, is moving either on a path of gradual loss of function or on a path of movement, maintenance, and improvement of function. The body operates on the opposite principle from machines. When it is *not used*, it wears out. Especially when illness or pain occurs, the tendency is to "favor" or limit use of weak parts of the body to avoid pain and failure which can lead to shame and ridicule. Even if dysfunction and pain are not present, we have a tendency to ignore effective body maintenance and efficient function until something goes wrong.

Once something has gone wrong, or we fear certain activities because our bodies are no longer "good enough" to achieve success and appear smooth and competent, we can become trapped in feelings of failure and inability. Our attention becomes drawn to what we feel we *cannot do*. "It's no use going shopping because I can't get around like I used to." "I'm stuck at home because I can't drive the car." "I'm losing my friends because I can't play golf any more." The focus is on the activity at which you are sure you will fail rather than on a series of activities that might help you improve movement and flexibility.

We are not suggesting that people experiencing physical limitations, or those seeking greater freedom of movement, can become exceptional athletes just by changing their attitudes. However, we are certain that what *you think you can do* will either seriously limit or positively support your chances for success at any activity, depending on whether you are stuck in your feelings of failure or are working on a process of improvement. If you are not *moving toward improvement* of body function and flexibility, regardless of your present level of ability, then you will almost certainly experience a gradual loss of the capabilities you now have and will never regain the enjoyment of activities you have given up or discover the pleasures of new activities.

Although it may appear that these issues are important only to those with serious physical limitations who need a wheelchair or a walker or have restricted use of limbs, they apply to anyone who ever feels he or she can't do something because "I'm no longer up to it." If it is difficult to climb a flight of stairs or you have given up bowling because of some ache or pain, then your physical activity and potential is limited by lack of attention and care for your body.

Once pain, discomfort, or fear of failure teaches us to restrict use of the body, you will *anticipate* this pain, discomfort, or failure each time you consider activity. The anticipation of failure must be erased and new confidence gained. The body needs to be retaught how to be successful at things it has forgotten how to do.

Here are the steps to take in getting going again.

1. Learn how each muscle system moves. Discover this by

minimal, easy trials so that you have a sense of how each movement is made at the most minute level possible.

2. Using the progressive relaxation techniques, learn to relax your body and identify how each area of the body feels to you.

3. Pay particular attention to those muscle systems and parts of the body needing improvement of function.

4. Design some amusing beginning practice exercises that use the muscle systems you want to improve without strain or discomfort.

5. Gradually learn how to reuse these parts of your body, building your confidence by doing tasks in private at which you are not likely to fail.

6. At an elementary level, take up again some aspect of an activity you want to practice again and become accustomed to the way your body approaches this action. Go slowly. Don't set yourself up to compete with yourself or someone else who may unintentionally shame you.

7. Keep going.

Much of the sense of shame and failure about movement of the body comes from the attention drawn to you during "public performance." Commonplace acts you once performed with assurance may have become awkward and unpredictable. Sometimes, even among family or work associates this pressure from attention drawn to your actions can be very great. So, the secret of learning new body awareness and movement is to begin practicing in private.

First, learn something about the physical function of the body. List the actual parts and systems of your body in which you seek improved function, for example, fingers, right hand; muscles in the lower back; nerve-muscle coordination in the legs. How much do you know about how these systems in the body work? Can you identify and locate the muscles involved—not necessarily by their medical names, but by your sense of how they work and move in your body?

To help you develop this sense, obtain a book with clear pictures of the muscle, organ, and nervous systems of your body.

There is no need to memorize the scientific names. Just get a picture in your mind and a feeling in your body of the various parts and how they move together. Think about the joints and how they work with one another. Identify the muscle systems by feeling them with your fingers and moving them as you are touching each one.

During your progressive relaxation exercises, get in touch with those muscles, joints, or areas that are not working well or are in the way of activities you would like to do. Describe each problem in one word: burning, tight, stuck, numb, sharp, missing, frozen, lost, whatever seems to describe the feeling. As you proceed with the progressive relaxation, when you come to these places, take an extra breathing cycle with each one. During this extra cycle, say to yourself, "I am . . ." and choose the opposite expression from the description you chose before. If you choose "tight" to describe your present feeling, say, "I am loose" during the breathing cycle, and focus your awareness on the specific area to be loosened, relaxing it as you breathe. If you had chosen "burning," then say, "I am cool and refreshed" as you breathe through that area, and actually feel the cooling.

Activities for Body Awareness and Movement

Each person's situation is unique. There are far too many possibilities for the kinds of activities one might undertake for us to try to describe them all and hope we hit on the one most useful to you. We have created some examples to give you the idea of how you can design your own program. Use your imagination and ingenuity to improve the flexibility and movement of your body.

Make a note of three activities involving physical activity that you would like to accomplish. Think for a moment about what is in the way, blocking your participation in these activities. Make a brief statement in your notebook about these barriers; for example:

1. I would like to play golf, but experience a pain in my back when I walk any distance.

2. I would like to enjoy more sewing, but experience stiffness in my hands and fingers that frustrates me when I try to do fine work.

3. I would like to drive a car, but lack of coordination in my legs frightens me.

We discuss each of these three examples to give you ideas about how to proceed with the items you have written for yourself. After you have read through these examples, work out a gradual program of new activity for yourself to accomplish the goals you want to achieve.

1. *I would like to play golf, but am experiencing back pain.* During your progressive relaxation, locate the muscles that hurt when you walk. Where are they? How do they relate to other muscles? What type of activity aggravates them? Is some work or family problem associated with the time when you feel pain in these muscles?

Back pain usually involves spasms of muscles that have been overstressed. There are two large muscles running down either side of the spine that balance the "sides" of your body. One side may be stressed, so you favor it, sometimes telegraphing pain to the other side because it must then carry a greater load. If you can relax both sides, they will regain balance and will not have to work one against the other to avoid your pain. Then, gradual rebuilding of your muscle strength without the spasm will give you new confidence and experience of movement without pain.

Practice the progressive relaxation exercise regularly, perhaps twice a day. Focus your attention on these back muscles. Imagine knots in these muscles becoming untied. Imagine the muscles becoming supple and loose.

After you have done this for several days and feel some relaxation in your back, involve yourself in a light exercise, such as climbing a flight of stairs, that uses the muscles in question. Never push yourself, strain or force any muscles. Move lightly and easily, assuring yourself that the muscles are moving well. Experience them moving successfully without pain or distress. Your *memory* of the old pain and distress is one of the major inhibitors of relaxed movement of these muscles. We want your brain to learn that this painful memory is no longer appropriate.

As the muscles gain new strength, you will be able to move freely without distress. If you stay with it, moving a bit more each day, walking, climbing stairs, etc., you will feel your body acquiring new flexibility. Practice some easy golf swings or some putting in your yard or somewhere in private where you won't feel foolish if your style is rusty. Get a new sense of moving in your body without the fear of pain.

The process of retraining your muscles may take some time, perhaps weeks or months, but take it easy. Allow your body to relax and your fears will subside. Your body can and will work for you. It wants to work well with all the inherent vigor it possesses.

Continue to do the progressive relaxation exercises as part of your program, even after you begin to play golf again. Keep that tension from accumulating in the muscles and your body will remain flexible and successful.

2. *I would like to sew, but my fingers are stiff.* Learn about the muscles and joints involved in moving your fingers. Discover them in your body and get a sense of the small muscle movements required for sewing. Feel them with the fingers of your other hand and see how each one participates in movements necessary for sewing.

During your progressive relaxation techniques, pick a word describing how your hands feel when they won't work for you—stuck, stiff, rigid—and use an opposite word—free, flowing, loose—as you say, "My hands are . . ." during the extra breathing cycles. Do several extra cycles on your hands and give them special attention.

Then design some games to build finger dexterity. Get some unpopped popcorn or a group of coins and spread them out on a table. One by one, pick them up and put them in a container. Take a small, soft rubber ball and carry it at times, kneading it with your fingers.

Gain a new sense of what you can do with your hands and fingers, working just a bit each time without tiring yourself. Don't put a lot of effort into "trying." Be easy and relaxed about it. Do what you can do and let your ability to improve come slowly and comfortably. Simply keep at it. Don't blame yourself or bemoan your inability at the start. Accept where you are and go from there!

When you feel dexterity and movement returning to your hands, select a simple knitting or sewing project that will not require much fine, detailed work. Choose something you can put together simply to give you the sense of successful completion.

Gradually, you can work back into more complex work and experience success all along the line. Give yourself time. It will be worth it to be able to do the things you want to do.

3. *I want to drive, but am afraid of leg coordination.* Start with learning the muscle systems involved. What does it feel like to lift your leg and place it in another position? What muscles are involved, and what is the sequence of events? Feel these muscles with your fingers and get a sense of when you move each one.

Describe for yourself what it feels like when these muscles don't work the way you expect them to. Is there any particular sensation in your legs or body, or do you experience lack of function without pain or unusual sensation? If there is a certain feeling or sensation, give it a name, then choose its opposite, for example, numbness—sensitive, floppy—controllable, etc. When you do your progressive relaxation exercises, use your new opposite word to describe these muscle areas.

If there is no discernible sensation from the area, but your feeling is one of frustration, panic, or anger at your inability to function, then do some extra cycles as you work with these muscles and say, "I am calm," or words you choose, to relax your anxiety about this limitation.

Then set up an exercise similar to operating a car. Start your practice after a general progressive relaxation. For instance, sit in a chair with a small box or book in front of you on the floor. Lift your leg and place your foot on this object. Sense what muscles are used and how to control them.

When you achieve easy success with this small object, find a larger one that requires you to lift your foot higher. Develop your ability to move your legs as you need and want to. Discover not only how to lift them but what pressure to apply on the box or book when your foot is up on it, similar to pushing on your car brake or clutch. Are these different muscles than the lifting muscles?

Take your time. Avoid constant measurement of your success or difficulty, just keep practicing.

In each of these examples, we can see the steps of (1) identifying the muscles and systems that need improvement; (2) changing your awareness of them; (3) setting up a practice game to regain movement and control; and (4) gradually increasing the level of performance.

If you can set up a program for yourself to move through these four steps, you can achieve new levels of flexibility and success in body movement.

Cardiovascular Fitness

Many people with chronic disease or physical limitations feel they can no longer exercise. Looking on their bodies as failing, they feel doomed to a gradual decline of vitality. This perspective becomes a self-fulfilling prophecy.

Vitality and zest are directly related to your body's capacity to utilize oxygen, the necessary component for all metabolic and physical action. As oxygen intake and conversion decreases, so does vitality and zest, apparently validating the mistaken impression that the body has failed completely.

Oxygen utilization is directly related to breathing volume and exertion. The amount of oxygen which can be taken into the body is a function of both the total air volume capacity of the lungs and of the resiliency of the heart/lung/circulatory system. Therefore, exercise to improve oxygen intake capacity should stimulate both the breathing apparatus and the circulatory system.

Dr. Kenneth Cooper, author of *Aerobics*, the most widely read book on oxygen fitness, describes the attributes of exercises that build cardiovascular fitness: continuous, rhythmic, involving the entire body (arms, legs, torso), elevating the heart rate, and increasing body heat (perspiration). Jogging, brisk walking, rope-skipping, and swimming are four highly recommended aerobic exercises that meet all these criteria. Many sports may be good exercise—for example, tennis, racketball, golf, or bowling—but they lack the continuous, flowing quality of the recommended movements.

There are four results of regular exercise: increased body flexibility (wider range of motion), increased muscle strength, greater endurance, and improved oxygen conversion capacity.

When many people think of exercise, they imagine only gymnasium activities are designed for building muscle strength. Although this aspect of exercise can be important, we are more concerned here with flexibility, endurance, and oxygen.

Although people experiencing physical limitations may not be able to walk, jog, or skip rope, many can swim. Others can begin some form of regular exercise, even in a wheelchair. We strongly recommend that anyone, with or without physical problems, include in the regular routine of life some exercise that moves the entire body as much as possible. Doing something every day, or at least three times a week, will remove the limitations for activity in your body and provide you with a greater sense of vitality and zest.

Increasing your cardiovascular fitness will reduce the risk of a number of diseases, increase your general vitality and well-being, and give you greater strength and endurance to do the things you want to do.

There is a simple way to evaluate your present cardiovascular fitness and to keep track of your progress as you undertake an exercise program. Many people like to have yardsticks to measure their activity along the way.

This evaluation requires no equipment other than a clock or watch and simply involves monitoring your pulse rate before, during, and after exercise. In this way, you learn the amount of exercise it takes to increase your heart rate to certain levels and how long it takes your body to return to its normal resting heart beat. These two factors are a general measure of your cardiovascular fitness.

Our objective is to perform a three-stage exercise that will tell you a great deal about your present exercise capacity. You can use the same exercise whenever you want to measure your activity progress.

Some thoughts before beginning:

- If you have a history of cardiovascular difficulties, or have not been exercising or moving much at all, approach any physical exertion with reasonable caution. Be aware of how your body is responding and don't overdo. On the other hand, please don't use this as an excuse to do nothing.

People who have not been moving at all need cardiovascular stimulation and will benefit the most from getting moving again.

• If your resting pulse is above 85, we do not recommend this activity. There is a wide variation in resting pulse rates (from the sixties to the eighties), and a high resting pulse is not necessarily dangerous but should be checked. We assume you are seeking medical counsel about your situation. We highly recommend the progressive relaxation exercises for you at least once a day, preferably twice a day.

• This is not a test or punishment. Do not push yourself. If you sense signs of fatigue or dizziness, stop the test and record your feelings, how long you had exercised prior to these feelings, and the like. Rest and resume the activity later.

• As a rule of thumb, monitor your heartbeat so that your rate reaches no higher than 200 minus your age. If you are 45, keep your heart rate at 155 or below until you have a surer sense of your body and its capacity. Again, this is not a contest or a race, but a check for your own information. Don't push yourself to achieve some imagined goal. You are not training for the Olympics!

• It is not necessary to finish the whole process the first time. Do whatever you can comfortably do and stop. Record your information, then proceed through the five minute and ten minute recovery recordings. Don't punish yourself because you took on too much the first time. The idea is to get a sense of your capacity, not to measure against others or some ideal.

Checking Your Cardiovascular Fitness
1. Make a photocopy or a facsimile of the Pulse Rate Evaluation chart on a separate piece of paper.
2. Before you begin the exercise, sit quietly in a chair (do not lie down) and take your pulse rate on your wrist or neck. If you wish, count the beats for 30 seconds and multiply by 2

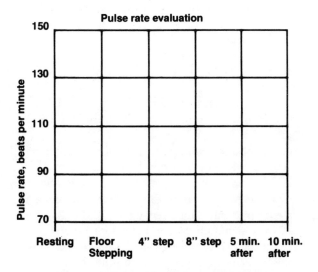

Figure 8.1   STRESS/STAMINA BALANCING
PULSE RATE EVALUATION

to get the 1-minute rate for recording on the chart. Enter this resting pulse on the first line on the left of the chart.

3. Get up and move about. Stretch your body and limber up by shaking your hands and feet rather vigorously.

4. Standing in a comfortable way, place your watch or clock so you can time a one-minute segment. By snapping your fingers, using a metronome or timer, or however you like, set up a 4-count rhythm at about 2 beats per second, 1–2–3–4, 1–2–3–4, 1–2–3–4, and so on.

5. During a one-minute timed segment, step forward on the level floor with your right foot, then bring your left foot up even, then back with your right foot, then bring the left foot back, all to the time of the four-count beat, like a brisk dance step.

6. At the conclusion of the one-minute segment, take your pulse and record it on the line second from the left on the chart.

7. For about a minute, walk around or stretch, do not sit down and rest. Keep your body loose and warm.

8. Using a box or board or some object about four inches high that will support your weight, prepare to do this same

262 THE KASLOW PROGRAM

four-count step exercise, this time stepping up on this object with the right foot, bringing up the left, back down with the right, then bringing down the left. Establish your four-count beat, time yourself for a one-minute segment again, and step briskly up onto the object and down again, this time using an up and down bounce.

9. At the conclusion of the one-minute four-inch step test, take and record your pulse on the third line from the left on the chart.

10. For about a minute, walk around and stretch. Do not sit down and rest. Keep your body loose and warm.

11. This time, use a stair or step that is about eight inches high. Do the same four-count rhythm, the same forward and back steps, but this time step up onto the stair or step. Time yourself for one minute as you have done before.

12. At the end of the eight-inch step exercise, take and record your pulse on the appropriate line on the chart.

13. Move around easily for about five minutes. Do not sit down. Walk slowly and swing your arms lightly. Now, take and record your pulse on the second line from the right on the chart.

14. Sit down and relax for about five minutes. Take and record your final pulse on the first line at the right on the chart. Connect each of the dots with a line across the chart.

You now have an initial measure of your response to only three minutes of progressively more strenuous exercise and of your cardiovascular system's recovery from this exercise after ten minutes. From time to time, you can repeat this evaluation and make a new graph. This will provide some good encouragement as you notice how much easier the exercise becomes, how you can exercise more with a smaller increase in heart rate, and how your rate of recovery from the exertion will improve in time.

Regular Exercise

If you are experiencing limited body function in some way, use your imagination to create some form of stimulating exercise. Get your breathing going and get oxygen into your body. Start with minimal use of the limited areas, but consider that you may be able to achieve full function again if you can generate a flexible, moving body. The whole process of regular exercise is important for you.

Deep breathing is the beginning for regular exercise, especially for those experiencing physical limitations. In the progressive relaxation exercises, you have been learning to breathe slowly and deeply. As a physical exercise, if you did nothing else, it would be of value to breathe fully, bringing air well down into the body, not just into the rib cage, for several minutes twice a day.

Also, do something—walking, jogging, swimming—at least three times a week. Think in terms of time rather than achievement. That is, set aside twenty or thirty minutes for your exercise and do whatever you can accomplish in that time. This may seem easier than setting some large goal, like walking or running a mile, and then fretting because that seems so hard to do. As you exercise regularly, your accomplishment will increase. Eventually, you will be doing quite a bit of exercise in twenty or thirty minutes.

One positive way to support your exercise program is to arrange for a group of friends who will exercise with you. The regular schedule and the support of others will keep you on track. It's so easy to let exercise time be diverted by other activities. But if others are involved, they will keep you moving and you will help in keeping them going.

Enjoy moving in whatever space you have. Skipping rope, dancing to music, or jogging in place can be worthwhile for those who do not have access to the outdoors. Exercise bicycles and rowing machines will provide good exercise if you enjoy the process, or try to find something you enjoy more.

SETTING UP AN ACTION CALENDAR

This workbook is designed to give you a general picture of the actions to be taken to improve your health situation by changing your choices relating to: (1) food rejectivity awareness; (2) general nutritional balance; (3) attitudes about your potential; (4) physical or mental stress recognition and relaxation; and (5) body awareness, flexibility, and movement and aerobic exercise.

Some of the activities provided are useful for evaluation, others for continuing development. Table 8.3 will give you a sense of how they fit together. Using this table as a guide, sit down with your calendar and think about the times during the day or week when you can practice these activities you have learned.

Table 8.3   WHEN TO USE WORKBOOK ACTIVITIES

	INITIAL TESTING PERIOD	CONTINUOUS ACTIVITY		
		DAILY	THREE TIMES PER WEEK	OCCASIONALLY
Diet Survey	xxx			
Resting Fast	xxx			xxx
Response Diet Testing	xxx			xxx
Diet Planning	xxx			xxx
Bowel Habits		Consider		
Self-Awareness Survey	xxx			xxx
Life Change Index	xxx			
Interaction Quality		Consider		
Stress Recognition		xxx		
Meditation/Affirmation		xxx		
Progressive Relaxation		xxx		
Body Movement Program		xxx or	xxx	
Cardiovascular Fitness	xxx	xxx or	xxx	

As we have suggested before, many of these activities can be shared in a group for more reliable participation and for support. Although the group will not do everything together, it is of value for such a group to meet once or twice a week to share personal experiences, to give each other support, and to develop ideas for further useful and pleasant activities.

So we suggest that you plan your personal health improvement program. Invest time in *yourself*. Only through your personal positive action will positive change be sure to occur. Only through your persistence and unwavering determination will you experience the pleasure of improvement.

We wish you well on your journey.

UPDATE: THE 8 MINI-FOOD MEAL PROGRAM

Our experience with the individualized Response Diet program has evolved into a very useful, innovative mode of eating for the individual who has developed a Metabolic Rejectivity Syndrome (MRS).

For the past twelve years, in our clinical research of MRS as a cause for a large number of chronic degenerative diseases not helped by the "usual and standard" drug therapies, we have determined at least three different manifestations of the body's rejection of foods.

1. *Impaired digestion.* Complete and total digestion is necessary for the body to utilize the nutrient qualities of food. In the MRS, food is not digested adequately and is therefore not available for metabolism by the liver and the rest of the body. Prolonged impairment of the digestive process appears to be a cause for the development of a number of chronic degenerative diseases. The patient may even be eating a well-balanced diet of the four primary foods in large quantities but with much of the food exiting in the stool undigested.

2. *Reaction to too much of one food.* In our research with the Response Diet, we determined that when the patient followed the single-food-per-day program there was evidence that eating too much of an "acceptable" food three times in a row caused clinical rejectivity. We then instituted a Response Diet program that consisted of a single food per meal. This allowed three or four different foods to be tested in a single day two-and-a-half to three-and-a-half hours apart. Again, a Metabolic Rejectivity phenomenon took place as a result of testing too much of a single food at one time.

3. *The processed food phenomenon.* Food that has been processed generally undergoes enzymatic changes that prevent the stomach and intestinal digestive enzymes from digesting the useable nutrients out of the food for the body's use. Chemical preservatives and insecticides cling to fruit and vegetables;

chemical fertilizers infiltrate the very substance of the food. These changes in the food substance can result in either rejectivity reactions or impaired digestion, if enough of such a food is eaten at one time. Since each food has its own nutrient value (although it may not be entirely free from pollutants or be a total nutrient), using a wide variety of foods minimizes the possibility of rejectivity or impairment of digestion.

Guidelines for the 8 Mini-Food Meal Program

The 8 Mini-Food Meal program successfully avoids the Rejectivity Response that occurs when the individual eats full quantities of three or four foods per meal and has three or four meals a day. The concept of eating small quantities of at least eight different foods per meal is actually not new or untested. Many ethnic groups have historically planned their daily diets using a wide variety of seasonal foods. For example, the Chinese meal consists of eight to ten small bowls of different foods eaten at one time.

Eating the mini-food meal way is easy and convenient. In fact, it was our patients who helped us devise the mini-food preparation system. In amounts sufficient to serve for three days, prepare six or seven different vegetables, a protein food (such as meat, fish, poultry, tofu, eggs, or beans), plus some complex carbohydrates (such as potato, rice, or millet). A person is thus provided with a wide variety of foods and does not need to cook small quantities of food on a daily basis. The food can be stored in the freezer for use in the next two days, after which another group of foods can be prepared in the same way.

Two to four teaspoons to two to four tablespoons of each food can be taken from the pots of prepared foods for each meal. Meals can be eaten every two-and-a-half to three-and-a-half hours to satisfy individual appetites and nutritional and energy needs. Some people eat four to six times a day and feel much better than they do on a three-meal-a-day program.

REFERENCES
AND
RESOURCES

Adams, Raymond, D., M.D. *The Modern Home Medical Advisor*, Des Moines: Meredith Press, 1968.

Ardell, Donald B. *High Level Wellness*. Emmaus, Pa: Rodale Press, 1977.

Airola, Paavo, N.D. *Are You Confused?* Phoenix: Health Plus, 1971.

Ballentine, Rudolph, M.D. *Diet & Nutrition: A Holistic Approach.* Honesdale, Pa: Himalayan International Institute, 1978.

Benson, Herbert, M.D. *The Relaxation Response.* New York: William Morrow, 1975.

Cooper, Kenneth, M.D. *Aerobics.* New York: Bantam, 1968.

Davis, Adelle. *Let's Eat Right and Keep Fit.* New York: New American Library, 1970.

Dufty, William. *Sugar Blues.* New York: Warner Books, 1975.

Green, Elmer and Green, Alyce. *Beyond Biofeedback.* New York: Delacorte Press, 1978.

Hendricks, Gay and Roberts, Thomas. *The Second Centering Book.* New York: Prentice-Hall, 1977.

Jacobsen, Michael F. *Nutrition Scoreboard.* New York: Avon, 1974.

Jacobsen, Michael F. and Brewster, Letitia. *The Changing American Diet.* Washington, DC: Center for Science in the Public Interest, 1978.

Leshan, Lawrence. *How to Meditate; A Guide to Self-Discovery.* New York: Bantam, 1975.

Leonard, Jon N.; Hofer, J.L.; and N. Pritikin. *Live Longer Now.* New York, Grosset & Dunlap, 1974.

Mann, Felix, M.D. *Acupuncture.* New York: Vintage, 1972.

Mandell, Marshall, M.D. and Scanlon, L.W. *Dr. Mandell's 5-Day Allergy Relief System.* New York: Crowell, 1979.

Margotta, Roberto. *The Story of Medicine.* New York: Golden Press, 1968.

McKeown, Thomas. *The Modern Rise of Population.* Norman, Ok: Academic World, 1976.

Pearce, Joseph Chilton. *Exploring the Crack in the Cosmic Egg.* New York: Julian Press, 1974.

Pelletier, Kenneth. *Mind as Healer, Mind as Slayer.* New York: Delta, 1977.

Pirsig, Robert. *Zen and the Art of Motorcycle Maintenance.* New York: Bantam, 1974.

Rand McNally Atlas of the Mind and Body. Chicago: Rand-McNally, 1976.

Rodale, J. I., and Staff. *Encyclopedia for Healthful Living.* Emmaus, PA: Rodale Press, 1974.

Rodale, J. I., and Staff. *Complete Book of Minerals for Health.* Emmaus, PA: Rodale Press, 1977.

Schroeder, Henry, A., M.D. *The Poisons Around Us.* Bloomington: Indiana University Press, 1974.

Tanner, Ogden. *Stress.* Alexandria, Va: Time-Life Books, 1976.

Tiger, Lionel. *Optimism: The Biology of Hope.* New York: Simon & Schuster, 1979.

U.S. Senate Select Committee on Nutrition and Health. *Diet Related to Killer Diseases V, Nutrition and Mental Health.* Washington, DC: U.S. Government Printing Office, 1977.

Watson, George. *Nutrition and Your Mind.* New York: Harper & Row, 1972.

Williams, Roger. *The Wonderful World Within You.* New York: Bantam, 1977.

INDEX